The Spiritual Dimension of

THERAPEUTIC
TOUCH

The Spiritual Dimension of
THERAPEUTIC TOUCH

DORA KUNZ
with
DOLORES KRIEGER, PH.D., R.N.

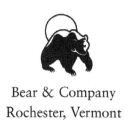

Bear & Company
Rochester, Vermont

Bear & Company
One Park Street
Rochester, Vermont 05767
www.InnerTraditions.com

Bear & Company is a division of Inner Traditions International

Library of Congress Cataloging-in-Publication Data

Kunz, Dora, 1904-
  The spiritual dimension of therapeutic touch / Dora Kunz with Dolores
Krieger.
    p. ; cm.
  ISBN 978-1-59143-025-4
1. Touch—Therapeutic use. 2. Mental healing. 3. Mind and body. 4.
Vital force—Therapeutic use.
[DNLM: 1. Therapeutic Touch. 2. Mind-Body Relations (Metaphysics)
3. Spiritual Therapies. WB 890 K975s 2004] I. Krieger, Dolores. II.
Title.
RZ999.K867 2004
615.8'9—dc22

                                                            2003027337

Printed and bound in the United States

10 9 8 7 6 5 4

Text design and layout by Priscilla Baker
This book was typeset in Sabon with Diotima and Delphin as display typefaces

Contents

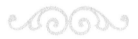

List of Exercises

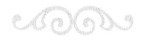

Acknowledgments

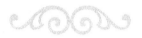

The initial idea for *The Spiritual Dimension of Therapeutic Touch* occurred in the 1990s with the thought that Dora Kunz herself would be writing this book. Other work intervened, however, and after her death I took on what proved to be a profoundly challenging but nevertheless thrilling learning experience. In the course of the project several persons stepped forward to help, and I am most pleased to note my appreciation of them.

Foremost, I would like to cite John Kunz, Dora's son, for his willingness to critique the manuscript so that it would reflect an accurate representation of Dora's voice and the significance of her work, and to share audio tapes from his personal archives containing Dora's own explanation of her unusual perceptual abilities. I am also grateful to both Pumpkin Hollow Foundation and to Orcas Island Foundation for making their audio tape libraries of Dora's recordings available to me.

Patricia Abrams shared with me her considerable acumen about the publishing world, and helped me plot out an initial outline. Julie Benofsky-Webb will forever be my heroine in this story because of her dependable and resolute volunteer assumption of the arduous but necessary task of typing the initial manuscript, as well as for providing me with the skills of an expert grammarian and being an astute sounding-board as she listened to my readings of the first draft. This necessitated that she ". . . learn all kinds of new things to accomplish this project"— as she wrote shortly after beginning to work with me—which I am sure will enrich her in her future role as a teacher of Therapeutic Touch. I also want to extend my appreciation to my adopted sister, Oh Shinnah Fast Wolf, who checked out the Commentaries for appropriate nuance of phrase as well as linguistic accuracy.

I am indebted to Charlie Elkind for giving us permission to include his poem about Dora in this book. He has captured the gleeful, high-spirited quality that characterized Dora and sensitively reflects the profound effect Dora had on her students. I also want to recognize Crystal Hawk's gift of the perceptive photograph of Dora and myself that she generously contributed to this book.

I would like to recognize the high caliber of professional expertise and sensitivity that the staff of Inner Traditions/Bear & Co. gave to the production of this book. In particular, I appreciated project editor Vickie Trihy, for her forbearing and kindly understanding of the vagaries of Montana electricity in (perhaps) finding its way to the Internet, and her generous support and encouragement on the occasional dark day when I doubted my ability to do justice to Dora's fine discernment and erudition in areas that to others remain obscure, inscrutable, and sometimes unbelievable. I also would like to recognize editor Nancy Yeilding's discriminating eye for the appropriate word or phrase, her ability to firmly grasp complex ideas, and her admirable background as a knowledgeable teacher of meditation. Mostly, however, I would like to thank them both for making the final writing of this book fun!

Finally, a word of deserved appreciation for the more than two dozen people who helped get the manuscript off the ground by each rough-typing one of Dora's tapes that had been personally meaningful.

DOLORES KRIEGER

An Introduction to Dora Kunz and to Therapeutic Touch

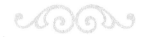

A Unique Approach to Healing

Therapeutic Touch (TT) is a contemporary interpretation of several ancient healing* practices. It can be described as the knowledgeable use of innate therapeutic functions of the body—which have rarely been fully realized in modern culture—to alleviate pain and to combat illness. It was my pleasure and privilege to develop and teach this healing method with a remarkable healer and friend, Dora Kunz.

It is difficult to categorize Dora Kunz (1904–1999), for there were so many unique facets to her personality. However, in brief, she was a clearly discerning and wisely compassionate world-class clairvoyant, who was born with these unusual perceptual abilities and chose to put them in the service of helping those in need. Besides working with this commitment in a brilliant manner, she had a delightfully contagious sense of humor that kept things in proportion in her daily life. Until the last years of her life she had a sharp, but facile, mind that was appreciative of the deeps of the Beauties of the Earth, and she freely taught others to value them too. Dora's tremendous insight into the transpersonal aspect of healing immeasurably enhanced the practice of Therapeutic Touch. This book

---

*Throughout the book, the term "healing" is primarily used to refer to alternative healing processes, rather than to conventional Western medicine. On occasion, the reference is to the general nature of all healing processes, which is made clear by the context.

conveys her exquisite understanding of this important dimension of healing—the spiritual dimension—along with a vivid sense of the dynamic and charismatic woman who brought it to light.

I was fortunate to collaborate with Dora on the development of Therapeutic Touch from the time of its founding in 1972. At this writing, TT has been taught in more than ninety countries besides the United States. In North America alone it has been practiced in over sixty medical centers and health agencies. Therapeutic Touch is considered a pioneer among modern alternative methods of healing because it is the first healing modality in Western history to be formally taught as an intrinsic part of a fully accredited graduate curriculum of a college or university. This occurred at New York University (NYU), New York City, in 1975 in a masters-level course called "Frontiers in Nursing" (E41.2363). "Frontiers in Nursing" continues today at NYU and is the model for similar courses taught at other colleges and universities in the United States and abroad.

For those readers who may not have studied Therapeutic Touch, I will briefly summarize its principles and practices here in the broadest terms. The purpose of this summary is to offer those unfamiliar with TT a glimpse of what this practice entails, so they will have a sense of the context in which Dora's teaching applies. It is by no means sufficient to prepare one to practice Therapeutic Touch. For instruction in this technique the reader should refer to my book, *Accepting Your Power to Heal* (Krieger, 1993). To locate available courses on Therapeutic Touch, consult the resource list at the end of this book.

Therapeutic Touch (TT) is a mode of transpersonal healing for people who are ill, debilitated, or traumatized. It can be used to relax the body, to reduce or eliminate pain, to accelerate healing, and to alleviate stress-related illness. It operates on the principle that the human body is an open energy system with innate therapeutic functions, and that this system forms energy patterns discernible to the trained and mindful healer. The focus of the Therapeutic Touch practitioner is the conscious direction of her own vital-energy flows or the modulation of the healee's energy field to correct imbalances that manifest as illness.

Briefly stated, the therapist begins the Therapeutic Touch process by centering, and maintains that state until the conclusion of the TT session. Consciously remaining in that state of consciousness enables her to access her own inner self during the TT interaction, an essential aspect of Therapeutic Touch that will be addressed throughout the book. Proceeding in that state, the therapist then performs techniques that sensitize certain subtle centers of consciousness, known as chakras in Sanskrit, which are embedded in the vital-energy field that overlies her hands. She then uses these hand chakras to evaluate the healee's vital-energy field for signs of imbalance in that field's subtle energy flows.

Based upon that information, she accesses other techniques for quickening or redirecting energy flow, as well as smoothing perceived disturbances. With considered intentionality, she uses her hands to specifically direct facets of her own store of vital-energy to the healee's areas of imbalance, or she sensitively modulates the healee's vital-energy flows, toward the end of helping the healee rebalance his own vital-energy field. Finally—still maintaining the state of sustained centering— she reassesses the healee's vital-energy field to evaluate whether appropriate rebalancing has in fact occurred, and to determine what may be done to further the on-going healing process.

Because the maintenance of sustained centering entails a critical shift to deeper levels of consciousness, the use of the TT process over time can give the therapist conscious access to profound realms of her own inner self. This permits her to operate with increasing awareness at the transpersonal level of consciousness during the enactment of Therapeutic Touch. It was Dora's particular gift as a teacher to be able to vividly clarify for the TT therapist the unusual dynamics of that transpersonal realm, enabling the therapist to engage the transpersonal aspects of Therapeutic Touch with clear insight and safety for both herself and the healee.

A Visionary Healer

Dora led a full family life and also was well traveled as a lecturer and a teacher of meditation throughout her life. She was in her middle years when circumstances first put her in touch with persons who were able to heal.* This happened during the course of a professional and personal

---

*For a brief but lucid account of Dora's early life, see Renee Weber in the Foreword to: Dora van Gelder Kunz, *The Personal Aura* (Wheaton, Ill.: Quest Books, 1991).

relationship that she had over many years with Otelia Bengtsson, M.D., whose specialty was in the study of allergies and immunology. Dr. Bengtsson often conferred with Dora about patients who had problems of a psychosomatic nature. This work honed Dora's skills of careful observation and gave her opportunities to study human relationships over long periods of time.

Dr. Bengtsson also introduced Dora to a number of other medical doctors, one of whom was Dr. Robert Laidlaw, then Chief of Psychiatry at Roosevelt Hospital in New York City. Dr. Laidlaw was interested in a wide variety of subjects, and one of them was alternative healing. In the 1960s he founded the first national medical conferences on alternative healing in the United States. These conferences, which continued for about three years, included a large array of medical doctors and scientists from both the physical and the life sciences, as well as several well-known healers and a variety of patients.

Dr. Laidlaw invited Dora to attend these medical conferences so that she could use her unusual capabilities to observe the interactions of subtle energies that occurred between the patients and the healers during the healing sessions. Most of the healings were done by the laying-on-of-hands and were performed within a religious context. Dora was present when the healers were interviewed by the doctors and when the healing sessions were taking place. She was able to describe the exchanges of subtle energetics, and she also could detail the dynamics of the vitalized energy flows as they coursed through the bodies of the patients. Dora noted these occasions as her first contact with healing and she was always appreciative to Dr. Laidlaw for opening the door to an interest that was to occupy her for the rest of her life.

Another strong influence on Dora's interest in healing was the work she did with a neuropsychiatrist, Shafica Karagulla, M.D., an associate of Wilder Penfield, M.D., of Canada, a neurosurgeon world-renowned for his work with epilepsy. Dr. Karagulla's area of interest was the study of hallucination; in fact, her original interest in Dora stemmed from her assumption that Dora's clairvoyance was a function of hallucination. However, upon meeting Dora and having an opportunity to study her closely, she realized her error. Within a short while they became friends, and later, colleagues, as they worked together on a book on chakras (Karagulla and Kunz, 1989).

Dr. Karagulla made arrangements for Dora to observe the doctor's patients without telling Dora anything about the patients' case histories or their diagnoses. Dora then observed the patients' vital-energy fields and the functioning of their chakras and reported her findings to Dr. Karagulla, who was on site also. Dr. Karagulla noted these findings according to a particular protocol she had developed, as she and Dora plunged into new territory in the study of human consciousness.

One of the aspects of the collaboration between Dr. Karagulla and Dora was their study of spontaneous healing, particularly that done through a famous charismatic healer, Katherine Kuhlman. In describing these healing sessions, Dora said that their unique aspect was that there was a buildup of vital-energy in the auditorium in which the healings were held. This progressive buildup of vital-energy occurred before the appearance of Katherine Kuhlman and was caused, Dora felt, by the often hour-long singing of hymns and prayers by the several thousand persons attending the healing sessions. The effect, Dora said, built a sense of harmony among the congregation, which augmented their receptivity to the healing session. She also found it very interesting that when Katherine Kuhlman did appear, she already knew that healings had taken place, and she could indicate the particular location in the hall where the healed persons were; she could say, for instance, "I see somebody in the balcony [which was a considerable distance from the stage where she was standing] being healed."

Dora described seeing "a powerful energy, which poured through her [Katherine Kuhlman], hit the person to be healed, and enveloped that person completely." Dora also reported seeing those people then walk unaided (in spite of their disabilities) to the front of the auditorium and climb the steps to the stage where Kuhlman waited. When they reached her, she extended her hands and blessed them individually. When the ceremony was over, the patients went before a board of medical doctors, who certified their healing. Dora also described angelic interactions that took place at the time of the healings (see Section VII: The Angelic Kingdom and Humanity).

Dora had a strong personal conviction—which, she was careful to point out, was *not* part of the conceptual system of Therapeutic Touch—of the validity of universal laws of karma that govern a person's destiny in reference to a very few large issues of his or her life. In the case of spontaneous healing, she clearly stated her conviction that the individual patient's destiny plays a large part:

In that instance, the patient's inner self [a term she used because she felt it to be more neutral than the word "soul"] takes complete command, and the healing is accomplished in a very few minutes. In other types of healing, such as Therapeutic Touch, the healing energies interact with the physical body, and the pain goes away, but the individual's habits that may have caused the pain are not completely eradicated, and the disease may continue in some form.

In addition to working closely with several people in the medical profession, Dora also worked with an outstanding healer, Oskar Estebany, who had taken part in the medical conferences organized by Dr. Laidlaw. Dora described Mr. Estebany as follows:

[a] fine and kind man, but he was not highly literate. . . . However, he was a great healer and never hesitated to help anyone who asked. He had a great simplicity and truly wanted to help all those he could. Mr. Estebany thought of healing and helping others as the central factor in his life. This was his basic reality, and everything else was at the periphery of his thinking. He dedicated himself to his healing work.

Dora and Mr. Estebany worked together at Pumpkin Hollow Farm, located in upstate New York, for a week or more at a time over a period of approximately five years, during which times Dr. Bengtsson and I were also present.

Dora described how she and Mr. Estebany worked together:

Whenever he was healing, Mr. Estebany had unusual abilities of concentration, and he strongly felt the healing energies that went through him. He treated people by touching them in different parts of the body, while conveying healing energies to them. However, he had little understanding about the physiology of the body, and he never bothered about where the disease originated. In fact, he did not have a clear idea of the healing process itself and he always took my suggestions about where to put his hands, whether to give light or strong energy to the patient and when to stop a treatment. We worked in that way for several years, he as healer and I as observer, and we became close personal friends.

It was during these healing sessions that Dora felt she clearly understood how the ability to heal could be developed. She taught me how to do the laying-on-of-hands and, as my experience and understanding increased, we realized that the ability to heal could be a worthwhile supplement for those in the health professions. It was then that Dora and I began discussions that led to our development of Therapeutic Touch. Dora has described this event in some detail:

Dr. Otelia Bengtsson, Dolores Krieger, and I worked together with Mr. Estebany for several years at Pumpkin Hollow. It was during that time that Dolores and I discussed, and then developed, Therapeutic Touch. None of the healers I spoke to would accept that we could teach any kind of healing to anybody. They said it was an impossibility, that healing can only be done if one is born with God's gift for it, and they were adamant about this. All of them said the same thing: "Impossible; it's not teachable!" However—based upon my interactions with the medical doctors whom I met through Dr. Bengtsson, and the nurses who were Dolores' students—I felt that it *would* be possible for people who were dedicated to helping humanity to learn how to heal. I felt we could work out a way to invoke their healing power.

Dolores and I went on to devise a healing method according to our own ideas, based upon our own experiences and judgments. She and I agreed upon a format; we set up workshops, invited health professionals to come and participate; and began what came to be known as Therapeutic Touch. We started to give classes at Pumpkin Hollow for persons whom Dolores was then teaching—masters and doctoral students at New York University who were also professional nurses. We chose to teach nurses and other health professionals because we felt that Therapeutic Touch therapists needed to have a sense of compassion and a strong feeling of wanting to help those in need.

Then, as now, we never paid any attention to the applicant's religion, race, ethnicity, and so on. Our first students had a broad background, coming from the megalopolis that is New York, where you have every religious, racial, and ethnic background imaginable. Our one prerequisite was that the applicants have a deep desire to help others who were ill. This assumption has remained foundational in our development of Therapeutic Touch.

We put before the students of TT the idea that we all belong to a greater universe than is apparent, of which peace and order are characteristic. We felt that there is a universal healing field that touches all people, and that having a specific religious belief was important only to the individual healer. Therapeutic Touch, therefore, is not based on a religion; it has no religious background. Until this day, neither Dolores nor I feel that the ability to heal is confined to one religious belief system.

Therapeutic Touch has proven helpful for a large array of illnesses. It has never achieved instantaneous healing, and that was never our purpose. But from the beginning we felt that we could develop a technique to help people to reduce their pain, lower their anxiety, accelerate their healing process, and get a sense that we all belong to a greater universe. An important aspect of the teaching of TT was the development of judicious verbal explanations of this interior healing experience in terms that could be understood by modern-day students. We have continued to refine and develop TT over the past quarter-century.

When we started Therapeutic Touch in 1972, we did not know that it would grow to have the worldwide acceptance it has today. We simply never thought about it. We worked with what was at hand and at what needed to be done. We never made far-flung, intricate plans; we gave Therapeutic Touch the freedom to grow through its own intrinsic expressions and goals. We did each day what seemed right to do, as we understood it, and went on. Therapeutic Touch has grown because the needs were real and unfulfilled. We started something that was in the spirit of the time; the opportunity was there, and we accepted it. We followed our instincts, and it constantly improved because we really wanted to teach those who were actively helping people how to add a new dimension to their work. But I don't think we thought Therapeutic Touch would spread so tremendously.

Over this quarter-century we consistently have given many workshops on Therapeutic Touch to several thousands of health professionals on both coasts of the United States and in many foreign countries.

To a lesser extent, we have also taught people outside the health field. TT therapists have been able to help many hundreds of people with a wide variety of illnesses. While absolute cure is rare, the conditions of most of these people have improved, and after a while they have regained their health as their own powers of regeneration have strengthened and their immune system has become more efficient.

Many holistic therapists have adapted some of the ideas of TT. They have changed these ideas, but I think TT gave them the initial impetus. Before TT was started, no public hospital would ever allow healing. Today, some are still skeptical, but they do not interfere with what we are doing, and more and more people are accepting it. How it will be modified, I do not know, and it really does not make a difference if it brings a new impetus. Let other people copy us; that is OK. They will modify it. But the basic ideas will remain, and they will be the same through time.

Dora's Collected Wisdom

As one can easily see, Dora Kunz led a rich life of rare experiences. The development of Therapeutic Touch—which, at this writing, has enabled the compassionate helping and healing of those in need to be accessible to countless thousands of people—took a great toll on her time. Her energies were boundless, so that was never a consideration, but she did not have the opportunity to fully state her wise and deeply insightful teaching on Therapeutic Touch in book form. In the pages that follow I have attempted to simulate this by transposing the spoken word to the written word, utilizing several dozens of audiotapes of classes and talks given by Dora on Therapeutic Touch over the years. In this, I have been, I am sure, only partly successful. A major reason is that one of the essential characteristics of Dora's means of communication was an inimitable and uninhibited, but decorous, use of body language to describe subtle behavior and events that are difficult or impossible to convey in the English language. They were appropriate to the occasion, but, unfortunately, inaccessible to audiotape recording! However, I was present at almost all of the talks from which I draw the narrative and therefore knew the contexts in which Dora's remarks were made. Thus, in the pages that follow, I can vouch that at least eighty percent is pure Dora . . . and admit that the remaining twenty percent is pure awe.

There are two aspects to Therapeutic Touch. One facet is of course concerned with the compassionate healing or helping of those who are ill, disabled, or exhausted of vital-energy. The other characteristic feature of Therapeutic Touch, however, relates to the inner journey of the TT therapist who is committed to healing those in need. The former is concerned largely with the development of an expertise in skills related to the restorative interactions between healer and healee during the Therapeutic Touch session; the latter concerns the effects that the Therapeutic Touch process has on the worldview and lifestyle of the TT therapist. In *The Spiritual Dimension of Therapeutic Touch*, Dora responds to both of these integral components in some detail in the seven sections in which the book is arranged. I have prefaced each section with introductory text to provide an overview, background, and context for that series of Dora's lecture transcripts.

The initial essays in Section I examine (from Dora's singular perspective) the concepts of the levels of human consciousness as they relate to the healing process. Of particular note are her discussions of how we can become more sensitive to the involvement of the inner self in our daily lives and how the Therapeutic Touch therapist accesses the universal healing field, as well as her suggestions for focusing the centering of consciousness in the heart chakra. Dora's very insightful examination of her own clairvoyant perceptions and her recommendations for the development of psychic and spiritual awareness are also of special interest.

The second section of the book looks at Therapeutic Touch within the context of process, particularly the concept of order in the universe, a universal law that underlies the patterning and organization of all healing and regeneration. Dora also discusses the unity that binds all Nature in close relationship, and is a distinguishing characteristic of the expression of the inner self in our lives. She suggests how one can become consciously aware of the sense of unity when identifying with the inner self. There is an impressive and thought-provoking consideration of death as a final transition of consciousness and of destiny, which makes each individual's life unique. Included are several exercises in visualization and meditation that strengthen the experiential understanding of these ideas.

It should be mentioned that Dora did not set up the exercises that are distributed throughout the text; rather, they were abstracted from the content of several of her lectures for the purposes of this book. It also should be noted that Dora's use of the feminine for the Therapeutic Touch therapist and the masculine for the healee or patient stems from the fact that most TT therapists are women. While Therapeutic Touch can be and is practiced by both men and women, that usage has been adhered to in order to provide more clarity about when the reference is to the actions or feelings of the TT therapist and when it is to those of the healee.

In Section III Dora examines the nature of the Therapeutic Touch process. An original insight is that Therapeutic Touch is not so much healing per se, as it is concerned with helping the healee to bring order out of the disorder caused by his illness. In this, she considers problems of obstructions to the healing flow, probes the relationship of emotion to pain, and clarifies the effect of the mind-pictures we constantly create. Particularly noteworthy is her discussion of the sensitive child—who is unable to dissipate his emotions and thereafter is deeply, and often cyclically, affected by them—and the manner in which memory designs our self-image.

Chakras and the Therapeutic Touch process are considered in Section IV. Chakras are looked upon as centers of various kinds of consciousness in the healthy person; however, their rhythm and consequent functions are disturbed in illness. Several clinical examples are examined and suggestions are made for appropriate Therapeutic Touch intervention. In addition, Dora mentions at least two ideas that are rarely discussed: the effect of Therapeutic Touch on the TT therapist's chakras, and the effect of that combination of events on the healee's chakras.

She then looks at the clinical problems of Therapeutic Touch within the context of wholeness in the fifth section. Much of this section is set up as suggestions for treating specific physical and emotional ailments. As she delves into the end-stages of certain conditions, Dora explains methods of supporting a person with a terminal illness during the dying process.

Section VI is given over to several questions that were asked during Dora's talks and the answers she gave. These are included in an attempt to fill in a number of byways that remain unexplored or were inadequately presented.

An intriguing aspect of Dora's unconventional abilities concerns her life-long high competence in communicating with intelligences in a parallel state of being, whom we call angels. I have concluded this book with a final section of Dora's discussion on these beings and her appraisal of them, particularly as it concerns their help during the healing process because—as is very evident as one tries to make sense out of our current world affairs—it is time.

DOLORES KRIEGER
THE ROCKERY,
COLUMBIA FALLS, MONTANA

CONSCIOUSNESS AND HEALING

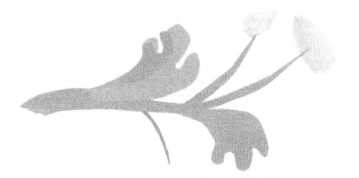

Introductory Comments

As Therapeutic Touch is both a technique for healing and an inner journey for the TT therapist, our aim in developing it was to teach it in such a manner that the therapist would not only be made aware of the more mechanical aspects of the healing process like the placement of hands, the use of specific chakras, and the projection of certain feeling states, such as love, and so on, but she would also understand why these postures or states of consciousness were being assumed.

As a background for such understanding, in this section Dora notes the central role of consciousness in the definition of ourselves as human beings, and that this consciousness has several aspects or levels. Importantly, she reminds us that—in order for these levels of consciousness to become fully expressed through one's personality—they must be filtered down through the brain, that is, in sensory and motor functions, and enacted in one's daily life. For the TT therapist this means that she must learn to use those levels of consciousness in her TT practice.

Since these levels of consciousness are enfolded around a central core of intelligence, the inner self or soul of the person, the therapist must frequently turn inward toward deeper dimensions of self in the consistent practice of TT. This inner journey of the TT therapist is basically concerned with finding out who one is, both as an individual and as a healer, and then engaging in practices to awaken in-depth personal growth in both spheres. This is realized by learning to consciously access the inner self to produce the necessary milieu of serenity and stillness as one acts as an instrument to help or to heal someone in need. The major requisite for this accomplishment is compassionate concern for those in pain, trauma, illness, or final transition, as well as a desire for involvement in inner work.

As a therapist undertakes the inner journey in learning Therapeutic Touch, she comes to see that the fundamental requirement is the realization that each individual is responsible for creating his or her own reality. If there is a particular belief system underlying Therapeutic Touch, it is that there is a background of order and intelligence in the universe with which one can make contact through meditation, sustained centering, or the fostering of a sense of identity with the inner self. Moreover, there is not only one, but multiple realities of which human consciousness can become aware.

The practice of sustained centering during Therapeutic Touch acts to change one's level of consciousness, for it provides an opportunity for the inner self to enter daily activities of living. This action reinforces one's ability to reach out to others with a sense of unition, and brings fresh energy to the healing act. In going out to those in need with compassionate concern, there is an expansion of the therapist's psychodynamic field, which serves to significantly intensify the degree of her sensitivity and to increase her awareness of the healee's needs. The TT process itself thus forces transformation to occur in the practicing therapist as she becomes more sensitive to the universal healing field and more compassionate to those in need of healing. This transformation may also lead to the acquisition of the capacity to sensitively perceive fine vital-energy states.

Although all persons have the potential to be completely aware of the full spectrum of these levels of consciousness, few are able to actualize this fullness in their daily life or in their practice of Therapeutic Touch. Unlike most of us who perceive subtle energies through the felt perception of non-tactile sensations or feeling tones during engagement with the TT process, Dora actually visualized the fine energies with which the TT process is engaged. In this section, Dora discusses her own ability to "see true," the actual translation of the word *clairvoyance*. Dora extends our experience by describing, from her point of view, the subtle energy complexes responsible for the body's vigor, vitality, and animation, thereby giving the reader a clearer sense of the incessant changes that occur in rhythm and timing, changes that one may feel, though not necessarily "see," while engaged in the TT process. She also indicates how the TT therapist registers imbalances in energy flow when a person is ill, and how she might further develop these sensitivities, a knowledge base that can considerably enhance the confidence level at which Therapeutic Touch is practiced.

Levels of Consciousness

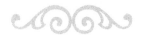

Overview

CONSCIOUSNESS IS A VERY COMPLICATED SUBJECT, but if we did not possess it, we would not be human beings; moreover, consciousness is central to the Therapeutic Touch process. *We rarely recognize that it is consciousness that makes us aware of one another, giving us the ability to interact, to think, to appreciate different events, to understand them, and to interpret them in our own way.*

I have had a very long life and have been able to exchange ideas on consciousness with many people, so I have had the opportunity to think deeply about human consciousness. Within each of us are various levels of consciousness in which we live and have our being. Taken together, these different levels develop from childhood onward and make up our individual personality. These levels of consciousness are: the inner self, the consciousness in the physical body, the emotional energy field, the mental energy field, the intuitional energy field, and unitive or inspirational consciousness. They are distinct but also intertwined and can all be accessed by the inner self. As I perceive them, they are common to all people but fully functional only in a small percentage.

It is very important to recognize that the human brain is the medium through which we interpret these levels of consciousness. They all go through the brain and affect it as the consciousness is transmitted to the physical level. The brain is a very sensitive instrument for the spectrum of human expression. Without it, we could not distinguish, could not think out, and could not interpret our thoughts and feelings. Although all these levels of consciousness are in all of us, parts of them are rarely used through most of our lives. However, it is possible to enhance our awareness by frequently thinking along these lines and through meditation.

The Idea of the Inner Self

Each human being has an inner self, a consciousness, at its highest, or deepest, level. *It is the enduring constant, the continuing background of all one's consciousness.* At birth the baby has, or is, an inner self, which is the central building force of the physical body. It is the consciousness that also extends beyond the death of the physical body and has often been called the soul. So many differing concepts have been assigned to the term "soul" over time, however, that I like to think of it as the inner self, a term that is neutral.

This inner self—our true self—is always a center of peace and quiet. When we get flashes of intuition or insight at critical periods in our life, we come closer to our inner self. But it is in meditation, more than with any other human activity, that we come closest to our true self.

Consciousness in the Physical Body

The physical body is the more material aspect of our inner self yet it has a certain level of consciousness of its own. It also has *vitality*, something we often acknowledge the importance of only when we are thoroughly fatigued. This vitality—which I call the vital body or vital-energy field—is a reflection of the order of the physical body and of the inner self. We are all familiar with the different timings and rhythms of our physical body. Our heart beats at one rhythm, our lungs breathe at somewhat different rhythm, and so on with the different organ functions of our body. The physical body also grows and develops according to its own timetable. It is the most complex time machine we know, but often we do not realize its elaborate complexity.

What is unique about the various functions of the physical body is that together they make up a marvelous, orderly system. Even though the organs are working at different rhythms, the body as a whole is working as a unity; it is this overall integration that makes for a healthy body. The intricate way the various organs coordinate and work together when they are healthy indicates to me that the physical body has a consciousness of its own. That consciousness continues to operate in spite of sickness or debility. Even as we medicate, treat, and help the body to heal, it is with the assumption that this underlying order will help to restore health.

Basically, the consciousness of the body is the information coming through the brain, particularly the information related to memory. The brain interprets the incoming information and therefore molds our behavior. Our interpretations are unique: two or three people may have the same experience, but the reaction of each individual may be different. Many people whom we see as patients are deficient or underfunctioning in the ability to use their brain and to think. In being flawed in this manner they often misinterpret many of the things they see and hear.

The physical body is subject to several diseases and malfunctions but basically it follows certain universal laws. The most fundamental law that every living thing adheres to is a pattern of birth-life-death. Nothing alive escapes it. This is a simple fact, which we often forget, particularly in the health professions. A baby comes into the world with a physical body that is already conditioned by a timing of birth, life, and death. Frankly, there is so much misery in this world because we simply do not accept that there is an ending as well as a birthing of each individual life. I think we should accept it, for it will make a difference in how we conduct our lives.

Emotional Energy Field

Next to the physical, one might say that there is an emotional level of consciousness, an emotional energy field. The subtle energies of the emotional level of consciousness or "feeling body" are different from the grosser energies of the physical body, but the two impinge upon one another. At the emotional level there is a sort of awareness of the energetic reactions of the body itself. And our feelings, without our being aware of it, affect the vitality of our physical body. Today even allo-pathic medicine accepts that our emotions impact our physical health. Imagine that I am angry; the emotional field sends energy downward that affects the physical body, particularly the hormones. Science agrees that this would impact the biochemistry of my body. However, it also invades the life-energy—called *prana* in Sanskrit—around each organ. Certain parts of our body are more sensitive to and take in more of this interchange than do others, and these are the organs and systems that are vulnerable to psychosomatic illnesses.

This emotional level of consciousness has enormous power. We are all closely connected. Aside from our experiences with each other, we have feelings about our experiences. When we express our feelings we are sending out energy. If you feel anger, for example, you know for yourself that you are feeling a lot of energy, and that you are often projecting that same level of energy out to others. If you feel peaceful, the energy feels more integrated. We also take in the emotional and physical energies of others every day as we encounter other people during the various acts of daily living. When you feel love or hate—two of the most binding emotions in life—you reach out to another person, in either the love or hate relation, and it is an energy that goes directly from you to the other person.

We are able to send affective energies to one another through a universal emotional energy field or psychodynamic field, from which the essential substance and composition of each individual's local emotional field are derived. When we are sending emotions to one another, we are also affecting the universal field, which in turn has the potential to affect the emotions of all humankind. Without going into details that are extremely complex, one could say that this is the reason why, when many thousands of people are feeling the same particular emotion, they can have a tremendous effect in the world. An obvious example is the special atmosphere that seems to permeate the days around special events or major holidays such as Christmas. It is important therefore to think not only of the effect our emotions have on ourselves, but also of the chain reactions that may be brought about.

Mental Energy Field

Interpenetrating between our mind and our emotions is another level of consciousness, the mental energy field. Our thinking aspect has a powerful affect on our physical health, on our emotions, and on how we view ourselves. Thought energy has the ability to consider an emotion that is being felt and evaluate it against a set of moral values or accepted norms of behavior. When you feel anger, for instance, you may want to do something violent. The impulsive part of you wants to put it into action but your thinking process wants to restrain that impulse and decides, "That is a wrong thing to do and I must stop." In other words, you think out the consequences of the emotions and you consider controlling them, so that you are using both the energies of your emotional field and your thought, or mental, field.

The level of your thinking is closely related to this emotional-mental interaction. There are two types of thinking: one is closely attached to your emotions; the other is more abstract thinking that is somewhat divorced from the emotional field. A different level of energy is expanded into the atmosphere around the thinking person. Here the relation is not concerned with human beings, but with ideas. There are always intermixtures, where one's emotions are somewhat affected, but not as powerfully as one's physical actions. I think of mathematics as the level of pure thinking, because very few people feel emotional about mathematics.

When people do mathematics, they are using a different sense than feeling. The mathematician may have the capacity to see only his thoughts—what has been called his conceptual field—during the times that he is thinking of abstract, mathematical problems or ideas. Then the connection with the conceptual field is through his brain and is not very associated with his feelings, since it has no relation to emotional factors. Similarly, a level of clear thinking is activated when you study philosophy and figure out its underlying concepts.

Stable, clear, and well-defined powerful thought affects the universal conceptual field, which then can influence many people, both far away and in close proximity. This can be seen in the several incidents that have been reported in the past few years of many people in different parts of the world—very often researchers and mathematicians—who think of the same idea or come to similar conclusions at approximately the same time, even though they have never met or been in conscious communication.

Intuitional Energy Field

There is another level of consciousness that is concerned with creative thought. We literally open ourselves up to ideas, and we get flashes of intuition. I call it an intuitional energy field. And what does that mean? All of us have had the experience of pondering about something difficult to grasp and after a while we suddenly get an insight, with a feeling: this is right! We have a solution and the certainty that it is the appropriate answer to the problem. This kind of perception comes from a higher level of consciousness than the feelings or the thinking.

The term "intuition" does not quite explain all the complexities of this level of consciousness. To understand it in an appropriate perspective, we must look to the inner self. If we get an insight, it is partly because we have come closer to the inner self. The consciousness of the inner self is usually blocked by our daily concerns, by the thousand and one things that occupy our mind. Intuition takes place when the energy of the inner self breaks through that block to reach us at the level of our personality. The dynamics of intuition are difficult to understand because they happen instantly. The energy flashes down through the levels of consciousness, leaving behind a sense of stillness that stays with us for a while. When intuition strikes, we do not question it, we feel it is the truth, and it invariably solves whatever problem we are pondering.

This ability is more pronounced in some people than it is in others and does not depend upon emotional feelings. Many people of different vocations are devoted to what they are doing, and they also have a singular ability for intuitive interpretation. It is clearly seen in inspirational persons like artists and philosophers who have opened themselves up to flashes of intuition.

I have talked to many scientists who have told me that sometimes they have worked for years without being able to solve a problem. In desperation, they put aside their work on the problem and go on to other interests. Then—usually in a quiet time when they are by themselves, doing something simple, relaxing, and repetitive, such as going out for a walk—they may suddenly have an insight into the problem that presents the answer they had been seeking. This is a classic description of how intuition works. From my point of view, I think this happens when there is a moment of unification with the inner self. It comes from a level of what I call unity.

We begin to draw upon this level of consciousness when we meditate. In meditation we can achieve a sudden sense of unity between all our levels of consciousness. In addition to meditation, some people are able to increase their ability to be intuitive by the committed practice of concentration or sustained aspirations. The chakras—the centers of consciousness that we will discuss later—may increase their innate radiance. In doing so, they often may give us a sense of the future, a sense of urgency. As a result, we sometimes get a completely new insight, a new definition, or a new description of how things work. If the chakras work very closely together in a coordinated way, we get more of these flashes of intuition.

It should be noted that there is a clear difference between true intuition and fantasy. Intuition comes in a flash of insight. Its realization—of the answer to a problem, for instance—is complete. Fantasy is fundamentally based on the patterning of the mind as the person relates to it on a day-by-day basis and applies values to his or her reality. Intuition occurs most frequently after a person has thought deeply about a problem. The intense exercising of the mental capacity forges a link between the brain and the inner self. Information comes from a different dimension or perspective and, suddenly, the person gets a whole, complete understanding, whether the initial problem was simple or complex.

The inner self somehow connects with our mental capacity and gets translated (for it has to present itself in language that makes sense to the personality) as a total message that has meaning for the individual. In addition, one also gets a different sense of time, and this gives one a different perspective. The final difference between intuition and fantasy is the absolute certainty that accompanies the insight. Because of this, when a flash of intuition presents itself and is acted upon, it is life changing for many people.

If you misinterpret the intuition—OK; in time you will learn to discern between true intuition and fantasy and that will give you greater freedom to live the sort of life you want to live.

The Unitary Perspective

Beyond the physical, emotional, mental, and intuitive levels, there is a further level of consciousness that perceives from a point of view of unity and order. This unified point of view of the universe is the highest or deepest level of consciousness. Although it may not be used in some, this level is in all of us. We can—at least intellectually and sometimes emotionally—experience a sense of unity with all living beings. When people meditate, they begin to touch or to act upon that level of consciousness. We usually think of all things as being separate, but through meditation—or when we are simply quiet and dampen our sense of personality—we often get a glimpse of a sense of oneness. These conditions help to bring about the sense of deep peace so characteristic of conscious awareness of one's inner self. When we lose the sense of personality, a sense of unity becomes available. Sometimes people feel it just for a moment, and a few who are profoundly and intensely dedicated feel it a good part of the time.

Many people have strong religious feelings that dominate their thinking. They have a sense of religious unity with God, a sense of expanding consciousness, a devotion to a principle very much greater than themselves. They also get glimpses of a level of the inner self at which the sense of unity predominates, and sometimes become receptive to intuitions about the future.

There are a very few people who at all times have a sense of unity, a selflessness of spirit, wisdom, and an active intuition, and are committed to serving humankind. They have a sense of the inner self that reflects calmness and peacefulness in their daily lives, and they radiate this sense to others. While everybody has these innate levels of consciousness, they are not usually developed, so these people are very rare. They do not have an ordinary sense of self. They express things impersonally and try to transmit the wisdom they have gained to all people. I think the great teachers of the world have had that ability, because they have a deeper understanding of the unity inherent in all of Nature.

This level of consciousness also has a different view of time. It is not linear time: the seconds, minutes, and hours that dominate our everyday lives. Saying that may have little meaning for most people, but it is true nevertheless. Ordinarily our thoughts and emotions are occupied with our daily living but when we connect with the inner self and its very different sense of time, we very often get hunches about the future, and of what we should do. From there we also may have a wide range of experiences that take us a step farther, but they are filtered through the brain and interpreted through the individual's personality.

We cannot bypass the importance of the brain in the interactions between the various levels of consciousness. It links us to the physical world; otherwise we could not understand or interpret our experiences. While there are levels of consciousness much closer to the inner self, we mostly only experience reflections of them, because our brain does not interpret these high levels of consciousness well, and our emotions, which can also block these glimpses, are not well controlled.

In meditation with a dedicated group of people of like mind, one can often feel the sense of unity. This gives one a sense of peace, which is shared by the other members of the group as well, and this acts to reinforce the sense of unity. Even when those involved in a group meditation don't know one another, they can often feel a strong unity with each other. The purpose of meditation is to expand our consciousness, and to slowly become aware that there are many spiritual forces in the world. This awareness filters down through our various levels of consciousness as our inner self is activated by our daily life experiences.

Meditation is not the only way; we also might become aware of these levels of consciousness through prayer, for instance. Some people are deeply religious and feel that same inspiration. A lot of these experiences are the same, but individual interpretations may differ based on how people are brought up and conditioned by life's events. But, the sensation is the same, and there is not so much difference, except in words.

Centered Healing

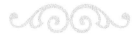

Meditation as a Link to the Inner Self

MEDITATION IS A KIND OF SELF-DISCIPLINE in which you are trying to harmonize the different levels of consciousness within you. There is a common agreement that there are principles of order underlying the dynamism of the universe, and that there are intelligent and energetic forces that maintain that order, even in the face of disorder. One reflection of this order is in the inner self that is at the core of each of us. There are many ways for the individual to get further clarity of awareness of the inner self, many different kinds of meditation practices, prayers, and other ways of reaching deeply into one's levels of consciousness. Therapeutic Touch itself has been called a walking meditation.

Most of us spend our lives in reactive behaviors, certain ways of feeling and thinking. Our emotions and our thoughts dominate the way we choose the reality to which we relate. We begin very early in life to respond to certain emotional and mental patterns without becoming aware of them, and these attitudes and moods strongly influence how we respond to life's events. While thoughts and feelings are part of our existence and can be influenced by an aspect of the inner self, meditation begins beyond the feeling-thinking level of consciousness in the arena of ideas and intuition.

In the meditation that is the starting point for Therapeutic Touch we deliberately focus our feeling-thinking energies in a different way. We withdraw the focus to a point within such as the heart center. We remain quiet for two or three minutes in order to realize that we have a center of peace and quiet within ourselves. We pull away from emotional reactions and impulses for a few moments to focus our energies in this inner way. Essentially, one says to oneself, "I am that peace and quiet, and the peace and quiet is my inner self." It is not said in those exact words, of course, but that is the general intent.

It is *I* who makes the decision to meditate for a few minutes each day. In doing so, the various levels of consciousness come closer to working in harmony than without that decisive, conscious effort. During this endeavor in the individual, a progressive process of physical relaxation takes place in the body. When properly done, one level of consciousness affects the next level. This cascade begins to reduce physical tensions and emotional stress.

Physically, the relaxation is of importance. However, if meditation is done for only a few minutes, just to relax the body by being calm and saying a few words—what many people think of as meditation—that is more truly a habit pattern, not a conscious effort. It is a nice habit pattern, but it does not have the same effect as when you say, "I want to achieve peace of mind and also a state of being in which I shall feel a sense of unity with others and with the universe, or God, or a greater consciousness."

If you have that intent and do a traditional form of meditation using ancient aspirations or the sacred literature of one of the various religions, you are focusing your mind as you say the words. In your mind you get a sense of peace, and it helps a great deal to start the day in this way. If you are meditating because of a desire to bring into your daily activities the uplifting feeling of reaching toward God or some other aspirational figure or symbol, there are then emotional consequences. If you started from a disturbed and inward-turned state, the effect can be one of breaking open or shattering those emotional patterns, enabling you to reach a state of expanded consciousness. There would also be an uplifting to a different level of consciousness than the emotional, and that would imbue you with a sense of unity.

One might think of this state as an expression of an intuitional field of consciousness. It would also affect all the other levels of consciousness. The effect on the physical body releases a new energy, and there is a sense of quiet that stays in the awareness for a while. All types of meditative practices suggest that you often find some sense of peace within yourself; it seems to be a universal finding. Concentrating on the idea of finding peace within yourself is a positive notion.

The idea of the inner self means that you think of yourself as strong, that within yourself some of the power of change is in your control. I do not think that all types of meditation stress that. You get beyond the feeling of just being relaxed in meditation; it is a sense within yourself of being deeply quiet and at peace, and in this stillness you are experiencing a sense of unity with the inner self. This sense of unity includes a sense of personal knowing that there is an essential kinship among all people, because we have levels of consciousness we all share. If we can truly recognize that we have these capacities, that these different levels of consciousness really exist within us, it will offer us a different perspective on how we can change ourselves and help others too.

The Universal Healing Field

There is a universal healing field in our cosmos; this seems to be the case since all living organisms have the capacity to heal themselves and, under the appropriate circumstances, to heal others also. An aspect of the inner self functions at that level, although we very rarely reach it with full consciousness. The two main components of the field are order and compassion. The description of it varies with one's individual experience and belief system. People in various religions call it "God" or "the healing spirit" according to their own personal interpretation or cultural background. I use the term "*universal* healing field," because, by definition, it cannot belong to only one interpretation or religion.

The universal healing field operates in Therapeutic Touch through the quiet moment of centering we do before we begin. All day long, as we go about our daily lives, we are interacting with one another, and taking in feelings, emotions, and thoughts as we interact. However, in that moment before we do Therapeutic Touch, we stop what we are doing. We center ourselves by focusing within, in our heart, and thinking of peace. What we are really doing is feeling the peace and quiet of the inner self. Once we have felt that, we project it to the patient. The moment of peace and quiet that we give ourselves to, coupled with our intention, builds a connection to the universal healing field, for we have opened ourselves to that field force. At that time we have integrated our levels of consciousness and act in a unitary way, as one piece.

Centering the Consciousness

Those who work with people—particularly in hospitals and other places where several sick persons are being given care—sympathetically try to help them by sending out energy to encompass and embrace the ailing persons with whom they come into contact. A nurse, for instance, may feel sorry for a patient and want to take away his or her pain, sadness, or troubles. This approach very often drains one's vitality. Centering is essentially the opposite approach. If you are truly centered, you are in touch with the universal healing field and can project its power. An important question, therefore, is: How can we, as healers, connect deeply with our own inner selves?

✿ Centering in the Heart ✿

Focus your attention in your heart and feel very quiet. In that quiet, envision a symbol or sense of your own inner self and dwell in the feeling evoked for a full minute. After a few moments, affirm to yourself: "I am that peace." In this meditation you will experience that within yourself there is a center of peace and quiet.

Staying with that feeling of peace, send your energy to someone who might need your help. In other words, project your thoughts to that person. Stay with the sense of peace radiating from within you as you continue your meditation on the stillness you feel in the region of your heart. When you have finished your meditation, take a deep breath and open your eyes.

Before we start Therapeutic Touch, we take a moment to be quiet and to center our thoughts and feelings in the heart. In that moment of silence, we try to dissociate from our own troubles and concerns and to feel at peace with the inner self. This ability of calming oneself is of utmost importance in healing others. If we can truly feel that peace for just a brief moment and open ourselves to the sense of stillness so characteristic of the inner self, then the energies from the universal healing field can be channeled to meet the needs of the patient.

When we do an assessment and try to determine what the problem is with a person, we are stretching our subtle energy fields and taking in, or being sensitive to, their energetics. We are also going outward when we heal, in directing energy to the ill person. When we center, we lessen the flow to the outside and go inward. Even without thinking about the inner self specifically, we can feel its characteristic peace and quiet working through us. This is not an easy state to maintain, but to the many thousands who practice it, it has become an essential feature of their practice of Therapeutic Touch and of their inner growth.

If you are quiet within yourself before you touch a patient or get involved in an emergency situation, then that center of calmness and peace protects you from taking in chaotic energy, even if you pick up the fear, panic, or anxiety of the persons involved. Having centered first, compassion will be directing your energy flows outward and simultaneously helping you to connect with the patient at a deeper level even before you begin.

You may be working with people in a great deal of pain, but you cannot work well with TT if you are only responding to the pain. You can be aware of the pain, and you are doing your level best to alleviate it using Therapeutic Touch. However, it is the centering that is the most important factor to have in place, and you will confirm that for yourself through experience. If you do not learn that, when you come upon someone who is suffering, you automatically take in some of that suffering. If you are centered, you will be aware of the suffering, but energetically you will not take it in while you work to help the healee dissipate it. Do you see the difference?

When you are centered, you do the healing from a place of profound peace and stillness and with a sense of certainty. If you are calm within, then you can encounter with equanimity another person's hostility, sadness, or any difficult emotional pattern the patient is facing. It is from this centered state of consciousness—which invites the presence of the inner self—that you can help the patient meet the necessities of his or her karma. At first you may find the act of centering difficult, but with time it becomes an ingrained way of life that can be called upon when needed.

Healing as a Natural Potential

Within reason, I think anyone can be taught how to do Therapeutic Touch. Some people cannot do it as well as others, but most can do it. Sensitivity to what other people feel is a sort of telepathy. I think almost everyone is telepathic to some degree and is able to pick up clues about whether a person is sad, for instance, or displaying more positive emotions. Not a word is spoken, but we pick up some of what another person is feeling. This is a common way of relating to each other that we all use almost automatically. We can more deeply understand our sensitivity in the context of the levels of consciousness in each of us. When we pick up thoughts and feelings without being consciously aware of what is happening, we are expanding our subtle fields and sympathetically reacting to other people's feelings.

The difference between healing and this sensitivity is that of willingly taking on a discipline of getting in touch with the quietness within you. Doing it mindfully increases its power immensely. You learn to work closely with your inner self for the purpose of truly helping a person, rather than just reacting and saying, "I'm sorry." It also helps you to remain unattached to the results of the TT. If you get terribly involved in the tragedies you see happening, you automatically will take in some of that negative feeling. Many people in that kind of situation feel tired or irritated because they feel they cannot do anything.

I prefer to work with nurses and doctors because they are used to seeing pain, and so they can be impersonal about it while they try to help. Most people will let their sorrow and sympathy dominate them, and they are overcome. If you begin to weep and feel very sorry you cannot do a good job. To be effective you need to be impersonal—that is, recognize that it is the patient's needs you are called upon to meet. That is why it is best to center your consciousness beyond the emotional level.

If you can stop what you are doing, even for a moment, and feel the quiet within, then do the best you can by calmly and gently sending positive thoughts, you will be amazed at how quickly such thoughts can make a difference in the atmosphere. Sending out a positive feeling in a peaceful way instead of dwelling on your personal shock can circumvent the negativity and help to bring forth positive aspects of the situation. It gives you another, healthier outlet for your emotions than just sorrow and a different way of looking at such situations.

In reference to the healing act itself, I think there are different degrees of healing. It is not easy for a person who is fairly new to it to put the concentration into it that is required. It takes practice to pick up the degree of pain and discomfort a person is feeling. When I watch students, it seems that they start to think about it, but do not really know how to heal, and as they try to bring in the healing energies, they "wobble." Slowly they get more of a sense of certainty in their ability and they can concentrate more deeply. If a person is really sick, and they take the time to put their hands on the healee's shoulders and along the spine, they can pick up a lot of the symptoms as long as they keep their minds open and unbiased. Doing this helps therapists to pick up pain particularly well; as they continue to practice and gain experience and confidence, the "wobblies" disappear.

If you are always asking, "Am I doing something well?" make up your mind that you are probably doing it better than you think, but you have fallen into the habit pattern of saying, "Am I doing it well?" If you are assured of your motivation in wanting to heal in the first place, do not doubt that you are doing it as well as you can. After being treated, when patients go home with the feeling "I felt a sense of unity. I felt better. Let me learn to relax and be quiet within myself and regain that sense of peace," that is a healing well done. We all want to make a contribution, and our inner stillness gives us the confidence that we can do so. It gives the inner self a way of expressing itself.

Healing and Therapeutic Touch are very complex subjects and difficult to understand. One thing you must learn to accept is that the patient's destiny is not in your hands. For instance, there are many millions of children worldwide whose destiny at birth—and "destiny" is the only appropriate word—is to have a terrible disease. I personally believe that each one of us has within us a consciousness that we experience at different levels as events in our existence. The inner self at our deepest level of consciousness has a sense, behind all our feelings, of profound peace and quiet and also a totally different sense of time.

You can help a person in many ways, but for the ultimate healing the patient must have access to plentiful energy. Through Therapeutic Touch he does have access to that energy, and it is in large enough amounts so that the patient himself can use it and determine his own destiny. If you treat someone and he dies, you can recognize that it was his destiny. Part of being a good healer is peacefully accepting death and pain, recognizing that these are natural processes. By being at peace, you can help a patient during the dying process and help the family, too. Your acceptance of death can help them to achieve a peace of mind that will remain with that family for a very long time.

The Role of Commitment and Compassion

It really takes dedication to pursue Therapeutic Touch, because it involves the study of a new dimension of consciousness. This is a large concept, but I think it is right to use the term, "new dimension of consciousness," because the TT therapists who are learning to be aware and to pick up where the sickness or imbalance is in a patient's subtle energy field are beginning to use a different level of consciousness.

Every time we center as we do in Therapeutic Touch, we create circumstances that allow the inner self to reach down to the ordinary consciousness of our personality. This gives us the flashes of intuition we receive as we treat people. Part of this effect comes because we are opening ourselves to become more sensitive to the subtle energies of the universal healing field. This state of mind is not difficult to attain when someone wants very much to help others.

We have taught many TT therapists how to simplify this process and teach it in a simple and clear manner. They can then go on to teach relatives of persons who are sick, and particularly those who are dying, to do TT with their ill relatives or friends. I have received letters from all over the country telling me of whole families, including children, who have been taught to do TT under such circumstances. This has given them the opportunity to touch their loved ones once again and to help the dying person in a peaceful passing. For all, it was a wonderful moment in which they had the opportunity to say goodbye to someone they loved who was in great pain.

I have now known people who have been practicing Therapeutic Touch for several years. I have noticed increasingly how they have changed individually from year to year. Their continued involvement in the Therapeutic Touch process radiates from them, changing their character and breaking some of their old habit patterns, often without their being aware of it. It is very encouraging to know that Therapeutic Touch has done that, and I emphasize it because you may not be seeing it from my point of view. Many have gained a sense of purpose in life because they are not only helping people physically, but also helping them access a new energy in a new way.

When a TT therapist projects healing energy onto another person, it also goes through her and gives her added energy, too. However tired the therapist is, when she does Therapeutic Touch, it energizes her. Over time, this changes a person fundamentally, giving a sense of inner direction that adds joy to one's life. Even though many Therapeutic Touch therapists work in hospitals and see terrible tragedies, the constant projection of healing energies integrates them and changes them. The inner self comes closer to the personality and the different levels of consciousness start acting together in an integrated fashion, rather than one at a time. This makes a great difference in a therapist's way of thinking and in her degree of sensitivity. It steadies her so that when things are difficult, those things that used to be disturbing no longer are.

As the inner center of calmness and peace is being called upon more frequently, it becomes dynamic and can be used more rapidly. The therapist, responding as a fine instrument, can now reach that incredibly large source of energy in Nature and in the universal healing field more quickly and with greater surety. An important part of being a good healer is the ability to achieve that sense of peace and quiet in any degree whatever. I have been with a lot of healers in my lifetime, and—even though their belief systems were different—they all shared the qualities of certainty and peace of mind.

The Expansion of Consciousness and Spiritual Growth

I think the search for spiritual growth that has caught the public fancy today is somewhat confusing. Today the search is for experiencing things for oneself. As part of this exploration, many people are meditating and they do experience an expansion of consciousness. I think this is a natural phase of meditation. It is as if for one moment within themselves they feel much greater than they normally are.

This stretching of consciousness—the experience of being part of a greater whole—takes many forms. Some people experience many colors. Others have a sense, for a few minutes, of belonging to something much greater than themselves. While spiritual growth involves expansions of consciousness such as these, true spiritual growth is accompanied by the certainty that one is an intrinsic part of a greater whole, a sense of genuinely wanting to help others, and an acknowledged commitment to give one's life to that cause.

Today people have varying degrees of this experience. However, sometimes what they are experiencing is not necessarily the idea that they can be of service to others. The word *guides* is mentioned a great deal, but to one versed in that world it seems they really are looking for entities—spooks. There is the sense that they are opening to all sorts of intelligence, and it gives some people a sense of personal power.

What is the difference between this and doing Therapeutic Touch? Basically it is very different to seek personal power than it is to have a desire to help, to be an instrument, which is my favorite word, or interpretation of what you aspire to. In trying to help another person, you get aligned with your own wholeness, your own spark of the inner self. In the process over time, you get flashes of intuition as you try to help the patient solve the problem of his illness. You are guided by the sense of unity with the patient when you remain on center, and by the conscious channeling of the healing power through the desire to help.

All healers I have talked to have emphasized that it is not they who are doing the healing; rather, they ascribe it to a greater power than themselves, a great impersonal power. That is much different than ascribing it to all sorts of spirits, guides, and so on. Therapeutic Touch stresses the universality of the healing force field, and most Therapeutic Touch therapists accept that, based upon their own experiences.

Spiritual growth should develop within you a greater sense of unity with whomever you are in touch, not a sense of distance or apartness. Altruism is the basis of achieving a level of unity with the consciousness of another. I think one also has a far greater confidence in oneself in this unitive, effortless effort to help or heal another and be of significant help to society.

You can also foster the spiritual growth of the patients you work with. Sick people often think of themselves as being useless, and this sense of being useless and dependent nurtures anger. Imagery often helps a person in such a state. You can ask them to image something beautiful in Nature, something simple that to them symbolizes being alive, for instance a flower or a tree. It must be something that they, rather than you, like.

Patients who must be dependent on others—who are helpless and have little to look forward to other than death—can also gain more acceptance of that when they are able to help others. You can say to them something such as the following: "Some people are sick for quite a long time; however if they are patient they can learn to be *listeners* to other people's troubles and fears. By doing that, they can be of service." We take it for granted, but by talking about it to such persons, some of their feeling of uselessness could disappear. Although they must lie in bed, if they can be friendly and project a sense of personal interest and concern for others, even for an hour a day for some weeks, it would indicate a spiritual growth, a hint that the inner self is becoming more aligned and integrated with the personality. They may go on to die, but they have grown in a spiritual sense because they have been able to give to others until the end. Their life has served a purpose, and they can go in peace. We very rarely think of that, but it may be the most important gift that a person can give to life.

Clairvoyant Perception of Levels of Consciousness

I have been able to perceive subtle energies since I was a child, and I am the fifth generation of persons in my family to do so. Throughout my life I have had unusual opportunities to learn how to use these abilities in considerable depth, and this has enabled me to keep these perceptual functions under voluntary control. I am able to see that there is a special life-energy associated with the physical body. This energy keeps the physical body alive. It surrounds all the organs and keeps moving through the body, somewhat like the circulation of blood, but at a finer, more subtle energy level related to the person's physical well being. This energy flow is part of the constitution of the physical body and it dies with the body. If a person is ill, this energy only extends a little bit beyond the physical body, whereas in health, it is vibrant, and can extend perhaps six or eight inches.

I call the subtle energy complex that is nearest the physical body and is the basis for its aliveness the vital-energy field. In this field I can see an outline of the energy patterns of the physical organs. While it would not be quite correct to say that there is a duplication of the organs in the vital-energy field, each organ does have a vital-energy pattern that is its own. For example, the physical liver is extremely complex with very many functions and the energy pattern of the liver in the vital-energy field also is very complicated. It has a direct relationship to the functioning of the physical organ, plus certain other elements that are very difficult to describe. Its functions are very extensive and difficult to assess, for it is not static; it is always dynamic, constantly in movement.

When I look at someone who is sick, I can actually *see* the illness. It looks like a distortion in the flow of the body's energy and a distortion in the energy flow around the physical organs. As I look at the pituitary, for instance, I can see the different energies. If a disease is present, there is a definite change in the characteristic energy system of the organs involved. Certain organs work closely together, such as the liver and the heart. Mostly the rhythm between them is very even; however, if a person is ill, there is a dysrhythmia in the timing of the energy flow, indicating that the body is not functioning well. When a TT therapist registers a cue of hot or cold while doing an assessment, what she is actually picking up is something related to the energy level of the organs and other tissues.

Interpenetrating the level of energy that travels around each organ, there are other energies that are of a finer and a faster quality. These are what we call emotions. More fine-spun still—interpenetrating both the emotions and the physical body—are our thoughts. Our feeling and thinking constitute the release of different kinds of energy that, in turn, affect our process of intuition, and so on. Although we all have and use these different levels of consciousness, we do not think of them as levels of consciousness, because they work instantly within us.

When I am observing an organ of a person who is ill, I am always impressed by the elaborate but elegant complexities of the physical body's multiple functions. I have to focus my mind in detailed concentration on the physical organ I am investigating as I search for the blockages caused by the disease process. Even while I am observing in this intensely focused manner, I also am aware of how the person's emotions are impacting the diseased area. The system that concerns simple feelings, the emotions, and thinking primarily about physical things can be called the psychodynamic field.

After I carefully note the physical effects of the person's unhealthy condition I look at the relations between his emotions and his mind. Then I may get a more integrated understanding of the patient's total condition. Having said that, it is important to make clear that there are times when the disease process itself can be entirely physical; that is, the cause does not begin at the emotional level, although there may be a reflection of the physical problem at the emotional level. I am distinguishing such fine points, even in this simple example, to indicate the need for detailed concentration when investigating the effects of the subtle energies of an ill person. It is challenging to do because the entire spectrum of subtle energies that constitute all levels of human consciousness are in constant flux and it is difficult to separate them.

Many people think they are seeing these subtle energies, particularly at the level of the vital-energy field. Most describe what they are seeing as white light. What they are actually describing is usually the periphery of the field, for there is neither black nor white in the field itself. The dynamics of these subtle energies are most accurately translatable as color, as pattern, and as a constant, restless flow.

To the observer, the vital-energy and psychodynamic fields appear to surround each individual. They appear ovoid, and seem to extend about eighteen inches to two feet around the physical body, the actual size being individual to each person. Every time a person feels some-thing, a color is produced around him at that moment; a vibration, so to speak, is set up throughout his psychodynamic field. The sum total of this is that the emotional atmosphere around each person is charged with colors that are especially patterned to the feelings that arise and are experienced or expressed by that person. Thus, a sensitive person could determine what the other person is feeling, and even what he is intending. The colors that I see around a person have both fluidity and radiance. The flowing effect is caused by the person's constant process of reacting, of ceaselessly responding to change. This movement goes on throughout the subtle energy fields, all of which interpenetrate the physical body. Because of this interpenetration, these energies flow inside as well as outside the body.

This is occurring in a dynamic organism that is constantly chang-ing, constantly moving. Therefore, one must realize that pictures such as those I have shown in my previous books are only representational; they do not give one the feeling of depth or movement that is actually taking place. They are diagrammatic only and so are misrepresentations of the actual perception of what is taking place in the vital-energy or psychodynamic fields. For example, if I look at a person's face, I see a solid mass of features, but the moment I try to see clairvoyantly or from a different level of consciousness, a totally different picture emerges. It is in constant flux, changing even as I am looking at it, as the moment-to-moment emotions fluctuate and are filtered through the brain.

I spent two years studying the functions of the brain and I learned a good deal. But I realized at the end of that time that I knew extraor-dinarily little. It is a fascinating subject from the point of view of phys-iology alone, where the nervous system is thought to be something like an electrical circuit. In terms of what I am trying to put before you now, that complexity increases a hundred fold. From the moment you turn on the sense to perceive a person's subtle energy system, you enter a dif-ferent world of perceptions, one in which it matters little what a person looks like physically. It has rules of its *own,* and you must give up your preconceptions.

Personal growth is indicated in the subtle energy fields of the indi-vidual in two ways. One is relative to the growth of the unborn child from the earliest stages of pregnancy through the subsequent birth and maturation of the person. Change continually takes place in the structure of the vital-energy field and in the psychodynamic field until the child is about twelve years old. Throughout the maturation process, growth of the physical organism continues.

As we go through adolescence other changes occur, particularly in how we perceive what is happening around us, and our actions and reactions to our environment and to other people. In all of these interchanges there is a constant meeting of aura (emotional energy field) against aura and a consequent ceaseless exchange of subtle energies.

It is during this period of individual development that we become self-conscious. As we grow into adulthood we begin to actualize the potentials with which we were born. If we have a sense of potential within ourselves, which is part of the divine, or the infinite, our responses to the interchange of energy with all that is outside of us take on a different, more spiritual or inner-directed, perspective that is unique to the individual.

In addition to all that I have told you so far, the vital-energy field has another complicating factor, the chakras. The subtle energy complexes that form the chakras function as centers of the various kinds of consciousness that express themselves through the human being. In this sense one could say, therefore, that the physical human body is the test object, or material, measurable reflection, of all subtle energy fields that make up human consciousness. I describe this assumption in considerable depth in Section IV: Chakras and the Therapeutic Touch Process.

On Developing Sensitivities

In our TT workshops I am often asked how one can develop psychic ability. I think it is sympathy and the willingness to be sensitive. Without being sensitive, I do not know how you could develop it. If you have been born sensitive to others, you can try experimenting with thought transference, and being compassionate and helpful to others, all of which will be useful in developing psychic ability.

Meditation is an appropriate tool to use to develop this sensitivity because the quiet of the meditative state gives one a solid, undisturbed foundation from which to work. While you are in that quiet state, you can go out in your mind to someone you know, with a sense of friendliness. We say, "go out to someone," and that is exactly what our energy field does when we direct an emotion to someone. The flows of our subtle energies "go out" to the periphery of the field, and the directive force of our intentionality conveys it to the object of our emotion, the other person. As we do this with purposefulness, the directed flow tends to change the patterning of our emotional habits as well.

The decision to learn to be quiet is a prime factor; if you are agitated, you do not create an atmosphere in which these abilities can thrive and your sensitivity can be strengthened. In my case I had unique parents, and my abilities were hereditary. We always had a meditation room, so meditation was taken for granted. My mother believed that children should start at five or six years of age by being quiet and getting used to being aware of themselves. This gradually developed into lifelong practices.

Very few people who are clairvoyant have the ability under control; they only perceive flashes of pictures or weakly interpreted hunches. Sometimes their emotional temperament leads them to exaggerate. If you want to be accurate in what you perceive, it is of great importance to check if your understanding is right. You have to have the moral courage to ask the person whom you are perceiving whether you are correct. If you never check up on your perceptions, you don't know if you are right or wrong. I think it is good from the outset of your training to find out if you are imagining things or if you are dealing with reality. If you do have psychic or healing gifts, do not preach at people.

The important issue in reference to clairvoyance is: what does it all mean? One should also ask: what did I learn from seeing the colors or images or symbols I perceived?

As people begin to learn Therapeutic Touch, they pick up cues during the assessment phase by feeling heat or cold or some other indicator in the energy field that surrounds the patient. As the TT therapist's hands come near an affected area, she feels a sudden cue that gives her a sense of where the pain is. Then the therapist thinks of the universal healing energy permeating that area of the body. Most frequently, this helps the patient's body to absorb the energy needed to deal with the pain.

For myself, I do not use my hands to perceive the aura. What I do takes considerable concentration. When I do put my hands on someone, I feel their tension, but I can also *see* where the disturbance is in their energy field. If a person has something wrong with their shoulder, for instance, I see not only the subtle energy field, but also I can pinpoint whether the problem is in the bone or joint.

When I was a little girl, I was not interested in the physiology of the body, but I could pick up people's feelings. When a person felt anger, love, or some other strong feeling, I could see the emotion in their subtle energy field as several different colors. As I grew up I learned to differentiate the emotions. Now I can also see the patterns one has built up—the repeated worries, the habits that automatically occur again and again, and other emotional reactions that indicate a person's basic character. I can also see the difficulties one has worked through.

In the TT workshops we have, I can see if the patients have been able to break through the patterns of how they think of their sickness. If you can get people to change this pattern, and to realize that they— their inner selves—are something beyond and different from their symptoms, they might be more willing to try something new or change their attitude, which would be the beginning of change.

Section II:

THE CONTEXT OF
THERAPEUTIC TOUCH

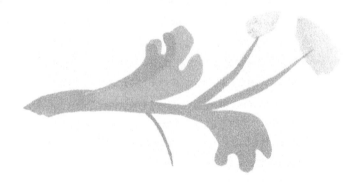

Introductory Comments

In this section, Dora reminds us that we each are an integral part of a larger universe, and that the individual being is a reflection of the ordered universe of which it is a part. The body itself is an organized complex of several orderly systems, each with its own intrinsic rhythmic patterning of subtle energy flows, wavelike pulsations of function, and periodicities of sequential growth and development. In a healthy individual these various facets engage themselves in a continual goal-oriented pursuit of renewal that appears to be effortlessly self-organizing, self-regulating, and self-healing. However, life-negating deviations from these systems in delicate balance occur in illness.

In the practice of Therapeutic Touch, it is important to be in continual remembrance that the individual is not limited to the bounded range of the subtle energies and realized consciousness. This larger recognition permits the therapist to be an unconditioned instrument for the unrestricted sweep of forces arising out of the universal healing field. Dora offers us the inspiring reminder that we can consciously implement the immeasurable abundance of energy continually radiating out from the open systems of Nature in the healing process. As one example, she discusses how the TT therapist can share the tremendous vitality of tree life. The vital-energies of trees seem to be curiously similar to the pranic forces that energize the healee during the TT process. That is why we often have a healee sit or lie at the base of a tree to reinforce the healing process after a TT session, enabling them to simply access the free-flowing vital-energies that enrich the tree's surround.

As Dora explained in Section I, the levels of consciousness of the individual interpenetrate one another in an orderly fashion. It is in sensing this interpenetration that the TT therapist realizes for a moment the totality of the whole person. Against this orderly background, the imbalances related to illness call themselves to the attention of the therapist during the TT session. It is the charge of the therapist to reintroduce that background of order and regularity to the body's systems by transmitting healing energies. In this way she helps the healee to regain adequate control of his faculties and to once more be calm, whole, and at peace. In so helping the healee regain integrity of being, the TT therapist herself—as the instrument through which this reintegration is occurring—also experiences an expansion of consciousness that reaffirms that we all are an intrinsic part of the essential nature of the universe.

Therapeutic Touch itself is essentially an act of quietude, for the point of entry into the TT process is a state of sustained centering. The maintenance of this state throughout the entirety of the TT session affects both the therapist and the healee. A sense of tranquility permeates the therapist's being, deeply affecting her psychodynamic and conceptual fields of consciousness. This allows her to work in a more integrated and focused fashion in the interest of the healee in need, and to open herself more fully to insight about that need. The stillness of the therapist tinges whatever energy she projects to the healee. The healee then absorbs this sense of stillness, much as we absorb the essence of love projected by someone who has great affection for us.

Being in an atmosphere of quietude fosters a relaxation response in the healee. This occurs quite quickly: the average time for a full relaxation response to occur during a TT treatment is within two to four minutes. Repeated studies have shown that the relaxation response facilitates immune system function, which supports the healing process. In addition, the patients of TT therapists who are able to access a deep state of sustained centering report that during the TT session they feel a sense of presence encompassing the therapist. This gives them a high degree of confidence in that therapist as well as a sense of enduring peace within themselves.

As a therapist strengthens her TT practice, she increasingly focuses attention in her heart chakra, which is the "home" of the inner self. In this way, the inner self takes a more active role in her daily activities, significantly influencing her attitudes and her interactions with others, stimulating insights into the consequences of her relationships. This affect is easy to project, enabling one to become a positive, constructive, and stabilizing influence within one's community. The actualization of one's potential to invite the inner self to be a conscious part of one's daily activities—and making those activities of a healing and helping nature—

makes the practice of TT a "walking meditation," in which a quiet mind is maintained while one is immersed in meaningful activity.

Engagement in such states of consciousness acts to significantly change the meditator's human energy fields, with a consequent reflective change in capabilities and in character. There is a quickening of certain abilities, such as intuitive insight into the problems of healees with whom she is working, and an increased certainty and confidence in her practice of Therapeutic Touch. She feels more integrated in her activities and inspired in her desire to help or to heal those in need. The sense of deep peace naturally acts to reinforce a personal sense of oneness and unity that is inherent in all of Nature. Concomitantly she begins to notice an expanding consciousness of the ten thousand and one things in the universe, and a selflessness of spirit becomes evident through her practice of Therapeutic Touch as transpersonal, inner work.

Two diverse examples will serve to exemplify this process of personal transformation. A person who is a very well known lecturer and author of several books on alternative healing wrote of her first experience with TT therapists: ". . . there was an ineffable quality in their demeanor that was highly unusual. And I knew immediately that if I was ever in need of help or healing, I wanted someone to be with me through crisis with those characteristics—whatever they were." I think this description reflects the deep concern, personal interest, and commitment to be present for the healee that distinguishes those of a compassionate nature.

The second example is from data supporting the view that more people have sought and earned graduate degrees and doctorates after becoming TT therapists than after becoming practitioners of any comparable healing modality. This speaks to the strong drive among TT therapists to learn more and more deeply because their personal transformations are pressing them toward more profound psychological, mental, and spiritual horizons.

As the TT therapist begins a shift to a broader perspective, her compassion for the welfare of the ill, debilitated, or traumatized persons she is working with arouses in her mind questions of why they are in pain, or suffering, or dying. In our culture we typically delegate the authority to answer such concerns to religious institutions. Therapeutic Touch—which has been taught throughout the world to students of all the major belief systems—does not itself have any religious context. We have always considered a person's belief system to be his or her private affair. However, in this section Dora compassionately responds to the kind of searching questions asked by practitioners. She discusses the concept of destiny from her own point of view, after clearly stating that her subsequent remarks are not part of the teaching of Therapeutic Touch. This conceptualization comes out of her own experiences and thoughts about the considerable pain and sorrows one encounters during one's lifetime.

It is supplemented by a very clear explication of karma, a system of belief about the bases of cause and effect during a human lifetime and, to a certain extent, deathtime as well. It is left to the individual reader to determine whether the content of this discussion is significant to his or her own queries about life and death as they relate to the healing of those in need. From my own point of view, Dora's insights into the dynamics of living and dying have been personally valuable in helping me to help others in a knowledgeable way. Her discussion has been included in this book because her remarks have been so contributive to the resolution of concerns of TT therapists and healees, as well as those of relatives and friends involved in the traumas, crises, disasters, and dying process of those they loved.

Nature's Order
and Meditation

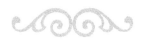

The Orderly Universe

IN THE PRACTICE OF THERAPEUTIC TOUCH, it is important for us to not only keep in mind the whole person—made up of all the levels of consciousness we have discussed—but also to recognize that each person is a part of an ordered universe. The concept of the whole person can be very difficult to visualize. It is easier, and actually more correct, to think of the concept of order.

There is an internal order in our make-up: there are many organs in the body, each with its own rhythm, vibration, cycling, and so on. In health they are all coordinated and work together toward the health of the body. The emotions of a "whole person" are well integrated and quiet; she has a balanced state of mind and is at peace with herself. A person who is completely healthy is living an integrated, orderly life. The order of the individual relates to the well-regulated and tranquil rhythmic progressions of natural processes in the universe.

The rhythm of birth, life, and death of the physical body is reflected in the farthest star, the whole orderly universe participating in a process of constant renewal. What we often do not realize is that nothing is still in the universe. There is an infinite, on-going repatterning taking place in which everything is going at a different rate energetically. In a true sense, the only constant in the universe is change, and this change occurs against a background of order.

Human beings are also in constant well-regulated change. However, the orderly pattern sometimes shifts for various reasons, breaking down into a disorderly pattern that we call disease. What you are doing in TT is bringing order, through the healing energies, to the healee. When you call upon a healing force to work through you and help a person who is sick, something also happens to you as the healer. You have in some sense an expansion of consciousness, even a small one, because you have been an instrument, and you have touched another person at different levels of consciousness. That puts you more in touch with the natural order of the universe.

Our Unity with Nature

By living in cities, more and more people have lost a sense of unity. We think we are a species apart, and become caught up in our thoughts and worries. Without realizing it, we unconsciously repeat these patterns of worry—which all of us have built into our lives—when we think of something in the back of our mind. The fundamental nature of these worries is such that they tend to interfere with true experiences of meditation, and they also block the flashes of intuition that lend insight into our problems. But when we go out to Nature we often spontaneously feel an underlying sense of peace. The rhythm of a rippling brook, or the sound of wind in the trees, or the cheerful crackle of fire in a hearth all carry that sense of peace and can positively affect our moods. Then it is easy to realize that we are part of Nature and gain a broader point of view. We become aware that we are not only in a place where things are green, but also that Nature encompasses the landscape, the seascape, and the skyscape of all of Earth and the living universe.

It is important to have the chance to recapture that sense of harmony and peace in natural surroundings. Then when we return to our homes—which are often nestled in artificial environments—we can draw upon that memory and it will give us peace of mind. If people are very lonely that sense of peace relieves the loneliness, too, reminding them that they are a part of a larger universe.

Whether sitting at the side of a waterfall or deep in a forest of trees, the effect is one of quieting. At the same time, there is the recognition that there is an enormous amount of energy in Nature. Therefore, learn to go out into natural surroundings whenever you can; seek out the vigor of a racing brook or stream, experience the stability of a mountain or a rock, or relate to a living tree. Respond to the rhythms and feel the strength that is available in Nature, and it will prove to be a source of new energy for you.

Trees as Symbols

We take trees so much for granted that we pass by their beauty and are unaware of their strength and vitality. I often think of them as symbols of grace and great strength because they have been in place so long and their roots are firmly in the ground, yet they reach toward the sunlight. In its lifetime a tree is shaken by winds and storms, but it goes through them and fulfills its purpose. A tree's life is closely analogous to our own. We are always reaching for the spiritual aspects of life while remaining rooted in our own ground, the reality that surrounds us. That helps us to remain stable while withstanding the vicissitudes of life. If we really *look* at the trees around us, they can give us a sense of belonging to the universe.

I always feel that trees have a certain consciousness of their own, and that when we sit among them there is an exchange in consciousness. They have an enormous abundance of vitality that they freely share, which is compatible with our own energy. In a general sense, I believe trees like us to be among them as friends. If you quietly say to them, "I appreciate you," or tell them how beautiful they are, their reaction to your thoughts will give you some of their enormous energy. In that way there will be a sort of communication between you and the trees. They like this interchange of feelings, and such an atmosphere of amiability and peacefulness will attract other wildlife as well.

We often suggest to our patients that when they are outdoors they should sit at the base of a tree and lean against its trunk to more easily assimilate its energies. If one opens oneself, the stream of vitality continually being sent out by the tree can be drawn upon, and that is deeply relaxing and quieting. If this is done frequently, one becomes aware of a feeling of consciousness from the tree, and it is a very friendly feeling.

This experience of the easy and pleasant therapeutic exchange of energies in the presence of trees can effortlessly be brought to memory at a later date. I find that to get rid of a very harassing thought, instead of thinking the opposite of that thought, just visualizing a tree, particularly one that I like, can effortlessly act as a substitute for the harassing thought and give me a sense of peace and stability. I sometimes think that visualizing a tree is the easiest therapy of all, for the relationship can affect us deeply and the memory of it can be of great help in times of need.

Visualizing the color green in a natural setting is also helpful. When you are at work and under stressful conditions, take a break for a moment or two and shift your consciousness. Visualize yourself in a forest, for instance. It would be so totally different from your workplace setting that it would provide a restful moment of respite for you, and help you to re-center your energies and start afresh.

The Quiet Within

In these very difficult times that we are going through, the capacity to feel quietness is most important. If you are in the health professions, you have the opportunity to reduce the negative energies to which patients are vulnerable by being quiet and not overreacting when tensions are high. Nurses, in particular, come in touch with a lot of sickness, a lot of sadness, which unconsciously drains part of their energy. A person who is quiet within and truly centered does not lose so much energy or take in so much chaotic energy as those who react to the stressed atmosphere.

However, very few people seem to be able to do this. Our minds willingly get cluttered with trivia, and in our daily lives we often get stuck in times of turmoil and forget that we have access to this natural power. When we have a problem, we get engrossed in talking about it. We get into a habit of repeatedly reviewing it, which blocks any insight or intuition from coming through. We can instead teach ourselves to be quiet for a while and thus open up to new insights.

No matter where we are, if we are willing to take five or ten minutes, look at the trees, feel the rhythm of Nature, listen, and keep our minds empty of everything else, the subtle beauties of Nature will become apparent to us. It is not quite as easy as it sounds, but once accomplished, it is a source of deep relaxation and peaceful quietude, as well as a sense of continuity. I always enjoy looking at trees and—more than looking—feeling a part of Nature and the cycle of living things.

⸿ A Meditation Exercise ⸾

Go out and for three minutes look at a brook, a tree, a mountain, or something else in Nature that draws your attention. Just for a very short time feel how beautiful and peaceful it is and let yourself feel a sense of oneness. This exercise can help you get used to using your mind to experience the sense of unity. Even done for a few minutes, it will help to expand your consciousness.

The next step is to begin to consciously focus your mind in your heart and say to yourself, "I am peaceful. I feel very quiet." What you will be doing is consciously shifting the focus of your attention to a deeper level. Then—thinking of your inner self and the energy of peace moving down through you—say, "I am that peace." When you are aware of that energy, it can give you a sense of strength, because at that moment you have achieved a certain unity with your inner self. These are the beginnings of the meditative process.

Stilling the Restless Mind

There is general agreement that there is movement in our thinking a good part of the day, whether we are conscious of it or not. Our minds are usually very restless and constantly leap from one idea to another. When you begin meditating, you will find that irrelevant notions can crowd out your desired stream of thought. You want to be quiet, but your other thoughts and urges impinge on the stability of your mind. Pictures and half-formed thoughts may race through your brain, making it seem a hopeless task to quiet your mind.

If this happens, I suggest that you do your meditation for only two minutes for the first two or three months. When you are at peace with yourself and have made even that short time of meditation a part of your lifestyle, then go further and deeper, slowly increasing the amount of time you spend in meditation. So many people start with the idea that they must meditate for a certain amount of time, and then basically get bored. Instead of setting out to meditate for a fixed amount of time, for instance, ten or twenty minutes, and then feeling guilty half the time because you are not concentrating, it seems sensible to do it gradually. I think meditation is something that one should begin in a slow way until one can say, "I love it, for I am quiet."

You will find that it is usually in the first one or two months that your mind will waver. If you persist and you are willing to discipline yourself, you can achieve the necessary quiet mind. First for two minutes, then for a bit longer, you will experience a profound stillness. It will give you strength as you learn to center your consciousness, focus your thoughts, and, finally, achieve a sense of deep peace. If you give yourself that time, you can understand the process that is taking place within you and enjoy it more intelligently, and—most importantly— you will be making better and longer contact with your inner self.

Bit by bit, the inner self will become unified with your feelings and your thinking. The more the inner self comes "down" and filters through your personality, the more profound the stillness you will perceive. Both the emotions and the mind will slow down and work together. The quiet will have a pervading effect, particularly on the emotions, and you will feel more truly yourself.

Visualizing Light to Focus Attention During Meditation

In meditation you are focusing your thinking. Sometimes, when you begin to meditate, you will not be able to focus on anything. You can help your concentration by thinking of expanding the consciousness. The sense of expansion is universal in meditation, but it sometimes lasts only a minute because the restless mind shifts to something else. To stop your mind from wandering, I suggest that you visualize your consciousness as expanding in light—a natural symbol of consciousness for many people. Visualization helps to focus the mind, and that steadies it. You will then have much more control and light will become an unconscious symbol of the inner self for you.

Meditation in Daily Life

All of life is a constant interchange of energies in which we continually pick up each other's feelings, whether we are aware of it or not. By meditative practices you can send out peaceful energies that help the environment. The experience of the inner self—the feeling that you are not only your personality, but that there is a center within you that can express calm and peace to a world that is suffering—will help you to realize that you are here for *practical* as well as altruistic purposes. If you achieve a peace of mind, knowledge, or insight, and send that out to people, it makes meditation a useful thing in daily life.

Most people wake up in the morning and immediately worry, "I have to do so many things. I have so many appointments today," and so on. We have a long agenda, even before we get out of bed. This habit puts a burden on our emotions, adding a kind of anxiety. Meditation offers a practical alternative because thinking of the inner self and then thinking of the sense of unity with all of life changes our perspective.

⁀ᓂ Changing Your Perspective of a Problem ᓂ⁀

If you can meditate, even for a few minutes, and gain a sense of quietness, of being at peace with yourself, your perspective will have changed. This is a good way to start the day. If you have many problems, think of them when you have finished your meditation, for your mind will be more focused and integrated throughout your levels of consciousness. You will have so much more to bring to the moment. Clearly state to yourself, "This is my problem," without worrying about it. I suggest you go through this process twice a day. The shift in perspective and consequent refocus of your consciousness will help you toward a solution.

Meditation will also give you a sense of proportion. If a difficult problem comes up, instead of immediately reacting or worrying, you will find that it is filtered, particularly if it occurs just after you have meditated. Both the anxiety and the anger that you might feel will be reduced. Your emotional problem will not possess you so completely when you can accept it and, in doing so, get a new view of the problem. Even though you are facing something that is difficult to solve, you will feel it or perceive it to a lesser degree because a quieting force from a different level will come down. You will begin to use not only your reason but also your intuition.

Many people are in a constant state of anxiety about events or about other people. Instead of surrounding those who are ill with healing, calming thoughts, they add to the negative energy that the patient is feeling. Our goal is to consciously avoid engaging in this constant interaction that eats away at our energies and distracts us. By diverting our own minds from worry or other negative thoughts, we can give the patient added energy for healing.

Suggestion for Picking Up Your Energy Level

During the day, when your energy is beginning to feel low and perhaps causing you to feel irritable, try to stop what you are doing for two minutes and meditate briefly. Relax and visualize a peaceful light going through your whole being. This will re-energize you in a positive way and focus your remembrance on the center of peace and strength within you. Then, if you have time, direct your consciousness outward, into that sense of unity, and feel that you are one with the universe. Feeling that kinship with all living beings gives you a way, a medium, to send energy out, for you are part of it. If your time is short, just send the sense of unity out to others who may be in need. The effect of doing this will make a decided difference in your sense of inner balance and equanimity, and it also will pick up your energy level.

At other times you may have to be in the presence of a person who is very tiring to you. I would suggest that you stop what you are doing, and focus for a moment on sending that person good will. What you are doing will help the tiresome person and it will energize you. You will change your own energy level in the process, for it draws upon another level of consciousness.

When you focus your attention in your heart, the center of spiritual energy, and feel its peace and quiet, you can send out peaceful energies or help to somebody in need. Even if you don't actually feel it, but you recognize and acknowledge that it is an aspect of your inner self that you are expressing, you will avoid reacting to your personal feelings.

Many people impulsively hug those with whom they are in sympathy, or they say, "I love you." That assurance is not of great importance. The most important thing is to give them a sense of peace that they can feel within themselves. It is remarkable how you can project this energy, which then helps people relax and feel that profound stillness as their own.

Meditating makes one's lifestyle more in tune with the inner self, opening one to a greater capacity to love, to be sensitive, and to understand, all of which are important in human relations. Instead of rushing in and perhaps doing the wrong thing out of either sympathy or dislike, you can meditate and still yourself. By taking a deep breath and remaining quiet within yourself—even if it takes two or three minutes—you might avoid reacting angrily or impulsively and choosing rash actions.

⋐ൕ   *Breathing to Let Go of Tension*   ൏ൕ

I suggest that when you are very disturbed, stop what you are doing. Be still. Take a deep breath to relax yourself and let go, really let go, of all tension. Feel that freedom from concern for a few moments and then slowly and fully breathe. The moment you get tense, you reduce your intake of vital-energy. "Letting go" and breathing fully helps your body come into balance again and regain its fundamental rhythm.

If you can be still for one moment, you might get an intuition, and you will know with certainty what you should do. Everyone has that intuitive level of consciousness, and if you can express it, you can develop and fine-tune it. Therapeutic Touch is one way of learning to do that, because you use your intuition to help people in a different way than is usually the case, and you do it frequently. As you experience your inner self over the years, you know that you can count on its strength; you become familiar with the quiet that marks its presence and the recognition that you are linked to an orderly universe. It gives you a different point of view. You come to see that many difficulties in life are a result of your uncontrolled, often impulsive reactions and are not necessary.

The inner self can work through all levels of consciousness and its power is beyond our usual expectations. Each of us can access the inner self in an affirmative way through meditation; we have the ability within our own self to learn to be quiet within and to grow spiritually. Meditation brings the experience of deep peace of mind, so that we can use the natural powers we have where we are in life at this time, now.

Once we have learned a little bit about meditation and the ways of quieting ourselves we should not underestimate our ability to help one another by sending out positive energies. These are our own senses that we project; they are not from outside sources and are within our control to use to help others, if we wish. If one looks at the historical record, even people who were ill have had the ability to accomplish remarkable feats.

A woman I met many years ago was a refugee from Russia. She had a terrible form of heart disease, with much pain. She was very frail, and had been expected to die several years previously, when she was twenty-five years old, but she lived to be sixty. She was very fortunate, and always acknowledged it, because she was married to a man she loved, and never have I seen a more devoted couple. He was a strong, healthy man, and their relationship was quite wonderful in many ways.

She became interested in meditation and—although she was very sick and in great pain at times—she realized that she had never been unhappy. When her pain abated, she meditated for long periods, and she realized that in this life her destiny was to have an incurable heart disease, and she accepted that. But she also realized that she was fortunate in having learned to meditate, because it gave her a peace of mind and sometimes respite from pain. When she died, it happened very peacefully.

Here was a person who seemed to have had a bad destiny. She went through the Russian Revolution, she had a long-time and painful illness, but she never thought of her own life circumstances. She felt that in her meditations she had found her path in life and her fulfillment.

She had a wonderful capacity to listen to people whatever her pain was, and they deeply felt her empathy for them. They opened to her, and it helped them to change. Even with a number of unfortunate factors against her, she nevertheless made a wonderful success of her life.

Her meditation and her marriage made her a secure person. She accepted her pain and her relationships were such that I would say that she was a woman who lived a truly spiritual life. The pain was physical and, of course, her emotions were involved, too. However, her other senses remained fairly undisturbed, and her intuition flowed through her. She had worked through the patience, the understanding, and the loving relationships, and she died having made peace with her personal commitments.

The point of this story is: do whatever you can to help others, *but do it*. Pick something that is within your ability to accomplish, and do that first. Then, go on to bigger things as they present themselves in life. When we started Therapeutic Touch, it never occurred to us that it would include thousands of people in so many countries throughout the world. We never had the slightest ambition about it; we just wanted to help. But it has grown beyond any expectation we might have had. So, start with small problems that are in front of you, and if bigger opportunities come, you will be ready. Although you cannot expect the world to change suddenly, make your small contribution, *but do it!* If you make the effort, you can compassionately and intelligently engage all of your strengths in the cause in which you believe.

Meditation Practice and Change in the Human Energy Field

If you can attain a quiet mind, you will become aware of a sense of peace as well as be able at times to pick up some of the tremendous energy in Nature. My observations of people who meditate regularly indicate that their constant practice significantly changes their human energy fields. I was once in a room full of people whom I did not know. We got into a conversation and I said to one of the men, "You have been meditating for many years," and I was absolutely certain of it.

Although outwardly he looked no different from other people, his capacity to expand his emotional field and the clarity of his mind showed me that he did something every day that was orderly and inspirational. He said, "Yes, you are perfectly right. I've been meditating for the past twenty-five years." The point I want to bring out is that to me it is apparent that there is a change in the levels of consciousness when people use their minds and emotions in an orderly way, and regular meditation is one way of doing that.

People who meditate—and also people who pray daily and do it with aspiration—may contact an inspirational level of consciousness. To properly grasp this, first we must realize that meditation, if it is properly done, affects all the levels of our consciousness, even that of the physical body. In trying to achieve this experience, the aspiration brings a sort of unity to the effort. The Dalai Lama is a fine model of someone who has worked to consciously realize this goal. I have been to India many times in my life, and I met him there on one of my visits, shortly after he had escaped from Tibet. He stayed for a few weeks in the Theosophical Society's headquarters in Adyar, Madras, where they had offered him refuge. He was the first outstanding person I had seen of that nature, and I was very impressed. Many years later, when I became National President of the Theosophical Society in America, the Dalai Lama was in our neighborhood. On behalf of the Theosophical Society, I invited him to visit, never thinking that he would come, but he did, and he spent three days with us. It was very interesting to me to see a person who carried such a profound sense of peace and quiet with him. While he was my guest, we had long walks together and talked about all sorts of things. He was interested in many, many things, but I never asked him one question; I thought I would leave him completely in peace and let him choose the topics of conversation.

He is a man who started meditating very early in life and he has achieved a great peace within himself; he has accepted his destiny. Of all the people I have met, the imprint of the inner self is expressed with his every action. He is also a very learned man, and his knowledge is profound, but he tries to be a very simple person. I am sure that if he talked about all that he knew, few would understand him, so he does not do that. Instead, he interacts with people at whatever level they are comfortable. To me he is a personification of one who has dedicated his life totally to helping humankind to have complete realization of the inner self. As he is a person who meditates a great deal, yellow is one of the colors in his subtle energy field and there are other colors, too, which indicate the fullness of his personality. There is a great deal of green, for he has great sympathy for people in need.

Also in India, some years ago, I met another unique man who impressed me, Father Bede. He became a famous Catholic priest although he was brought up as an intellectual and attended Oxford. He had great devotion, coupled with a first-class intellect, which is not a common combination. He was constantly praying, and he had achieved a profound inner strength, but he was also thinking deeply.

It would not be possible to live more simply than he did. He had reduced his life to the barest necessities. We talked sitting on the floor, all of us, eating very simple food and sleeping on wooden bunks. He said mass every day, and he did it with immense devotion. His congregation, which was small, was made up of poor and uneducated Indians. They followed their own religious traditions, but they came regularly and listened to his Christian mass. Some became Christians, others did not, but they were all drawn to this man. There were also Western people there, and some were famous scientists. All of them sat absolutely still and there was complete harmony between them. He said the mass, but he realized that Hinduism had also a great deal to contribute. He was unique in that way. Many of his listeners were Hindus, so he brought some of the ideas of Hinduism into what he said.

He was practicing deep meditation daily and—as in the man I mentioned previously—I could see the changes it had made in his consciousness. He shared his tremendous sense of insight and uplift. He had strong intuitive feelings, which he could transmit to an audience who were foreign to his background. He was able to convey his beliefs because he had the sense that there is a unity behind all humanity, and he related it to his religious belief. He could reach out to others, in sensitivity and intuition, and speak in terms they would understand, and he could appreciate other points of view.

Developing a Sense of Unity

The people who know how to truly meditate, like Father Bede and the Dalai Lama, can focus on their meditations for very long periods of time, because under those circumstances time makes no difference; it is irrelevant. For most people in the West, five to twenty minutes is the span in which they can pay full attention to their meditation. Some people have difficultly achieving even five minutes of concentrated meditation. Nevertheless, if you can focus full attention for five minutes, it can have a powerful effect on you. However, if you say the words but your attention is elsewhere, it has very little effect. It will have a general calming effect, but you will not reach that state of consciousness where for one moment, you deeply feel a sense of unity. If you sincerely meditate, it is an enormously energizing proceeding because you reach out to an expansion of consciousness and in the process there is an ingathering of fresh vital-energy.

When you have experienced this sense of unity, this expansion of consciousness, it can stimulate your mind, too. Many people are of the impression that the goal of meditation is to shut out the mind. This makes little sense because a powerful energy is experienced when you reach the intuitional level of consciousness and beyond that. Suddenly you have an intuitive flash, and you have the strength to do what you think is right, even against opposition. For one full moment you have the recognition: *I am doing that.* You have a sense of your own inner strength, and you are completely certain within yourself. When this happens, you have unified your various levels of consciousness with your inner self, at least for a moment.

The sense of unity is actually a great force that can release creative ideas—which may be distinctly perceivable—in the individual who keeps at it. Meditation can unleash this within as the intuitional level is reached, and so it becomes a discipline, a very important discipline. In a religious sense, you are reaching toward God. From a non-religious point of view, you are expanding your mind to the same content, but you would say that you are experiencing a sense of absolute unity. They are different expressions, but similar experiences.

If this happens—even a short moment of reaching the sense of being one with the universe—it energizes you powerfully. That expansion significantly affects the various levels of consciousness. There is a feeling of deep certainty about this sense of unity; nevertheless, small uncertainties may remain around the fringes, so to speak. Minor diversities may persist within this over-all unity. The effects of meditation are such that when you need it, it gives you a focus of enlightenment about these diversities. For instance, if you have a great interest, and if you can reach that unified state of mind, it will give you access to flashes of intuition about the things you want to know and understand.

However, you cannot sit still and simply say, "I am very interested in this; I want to have an intuition." That is one way of killing the opportunity for insight. Instead, think about it and feel it deep in your emotions. Be very still—the more still, the better—and then reach out to whatever interests you. It will come to you when you are ready for it, when you yourself are in a unified state of mind, without the demand: *I want it!* That "*I*" with which you identify yourself wants so many things, and it puts the emphasis on your emotions. The only way to draw upon the higher or deeper levels of consciousness with reliability is to transcend that instinctual identification and approach the sense of unity with a clear consciousness. It happens, all of a sudden, because you are prepared.

Destiny and Death

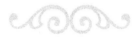

The Complexity of Time

BIRTH, LIFE, AND DEATH HAPPEN TO EVERY LIVING THING in the universe, from the life of the furthest star to the life of the smallest microbe. This is a law of Nature. It is important for those in the health professions to accept that no mere human can reverse this universal cycle. If a person can accept that view of life, it enables him or her to help a great many people with a sense of equanimity, with a better acceptance of whatever healing events follow.

My own insights have been gleaned by working with numerous people in divergent stages of health and disease, from my own personal clairvoyant experiences, and from the ancient literature. Everybody is born and eventually dies; this we take for granted. The aspect we will explore is: what is it within ourselves that experiences these ever-changing patterns of life?

I should point out that *what I am about to say is not part of Therapeutic Touch teaching*, but is what I personally believe: the inner self survives as a consciousness after death, and is the nucleus for the reentry into the life process. In each individual, the inner self comes into physical existence with a very few definite opportunities that are its destiny to fulfill. However, these events are not worked out in detail. If one accepts the idea of an inner self, the concept of karma—what I have called destiny—is logical.

From the point of view of the inner self, destiny and time do not have the same meaning. To us, time is so all-important. But the inner self has lived before and, I believe, will live again, after death; from that point of view, time has no meaning as we understand it. The inner self reflects both our past and our future; it is the part of us that contains the seeds and memories of past existences. Sometimes we meet someone and instantly feel at home with her, and a strong, lasting friendship blooms and endures. The strength of this friendship can be stronger than the ties we have with family members. From my point of view, this is karma, or destiny, at work. True bonding has nothing to do with our gender, parents, or other physical relationships of a lifetime; true bonding takes place at a deeper level, from self to self, and the roles we play from one lifetime to another may vary a great deal. The reason why we do not repeat the same roles each lifetime is that we need to learn new experiences. However, the "real" feeling we have for those we deeply love will be repeated, of that we can be sure. In some instances a parent may feel a stronger link with one child than another, and sometimes this relates to the links the two beings have had in former lives.

The family we are born into, even the time of birth, is somewhat predestined. Certain events in our lives, significant people we meet along the way, even the circumstances of our death, fit this category of predestination. The context in which I use the term *predestination* is in reference to certain tasks or accomplishments that need to be dealt with in this lifetime. Our tasks are incorporated into our life cycle. In the long run, years do not really matter; of more significance is the carry-through of these individualized tasks and accomplishments. Many people have precognitive dreams. As noted, the inner self has a very different sense of time, one that may be thought of as duration, rather than man-made tick-tock time. Because of this it knows and can present things, particularly major happenings in one's life, ahead of time. But this does not mean that everything is predestined.

When the inner self comes into a relationship with the fetus, that indicates that it has accepted certain limitations or conditions that will impact the person until death. There are not many conditions—perhaps four or five—but the limitations that do mark an individual's life are not accidental. The inner self has accepted those conditions in full awareness, and the individual works them out throughout life. All other events in that life are free or unconditioned, and how the person uses them is a personal decision.

This is an important idea to remember. Many babies are born with different kinds of illnesses or disabilities and one might say it is an unfair world, for they are brought into this world greatly handicapped by circumstances beyond their control. From my point of view, it is the inner self that has accepted that limitation as a condition for conscious development. Many people who are born in difficult circumstances work their problems out. Several escape formidable experiences and terrible setbacks by their own efforts because they have within themselves a drive to overcome their difficulties. They may go on to achieve great things, relating to incidents as challenges and opportunities to learn about their links to their own inner self. The inner self can work through all levels of consciousness; if you look at history, people with all kinds of illnesses have transcended them and gone on to do wonderful things.

An example of this concerns a girl I knew who came to this country to be medically helped. She had an incurable disease from early childhood onward, which, I believe, was predestined. It colored her whole life. In spite of medical intervention, she was never without pain for the twenty-five or more years that I knew her. However, she was adopted by an American, which enabled her to stay in this country. That made a tremendous difference in what subsequently happened to her. How she accepted her basic illness and all its progression and what she did under those circumstances was up to her.

All her life, she suffered pain and many limitations imposed by the nature of her illness. When I first knew her, the doctors said she would live a very short time, but she lived thirty-seven years beyond that. She was also subjected to many surgeries and hospitalizations, but her attitude was never negative. When people asked her how she was, she always cheerfully said, "Fine." She did not want people to feel anguished because of her. That, without doubt, was a life of suffering, but she had the joy of having many close friends, and wherever she went she was greeted with pleasure.

She said she wanted to be part of life and contribute like other people do and not get stuck in things she could do nothing about. She lived as fully as she could and she had the courage to look forward to tomorrow, never giving in unduly to periods of depression. One thing she could control was her attitude toward life events, and there she was determined to keep her freedom. She helped a lot of people by her example, not because she wanted to be an example but because she wanted to help people out of her compassion. She befriended many people, listened to their problems, and helped them in whatever way was feasible. This made her happy and gave her life meaning, even though she was under great limitations that were predestined.

She acted in others' behalf in the one way open to her—spiritually—and in many ways she gained a lot in spiritual development. Although she was severely restricted physically, she consciously changed her life, instead of doing nothing or bewailing her fate. In this way, through her conscious effort, she was able to transcend aspects of her destiny. Her example illustrates how important it is to encourage people to contribute even in little ways, even in the world of constant physical pain. This enables such people to draw upon the inner self and gives them opportunities to grow.

In this context, it is also important to realize that the sickness was not imposed without the assent of the inner self. From my perspective, some diseases are hard to cure when they deeply involve the person's karma. In some cases we can help to reduce the pain with Therapeutic Touch, but the disease process may continue.

At the same time, we have to keep in mind that just because a person gets an illness, it does not mean that they cannot get cured. Today the majority of illnesses can be helped. Children seem to be helped most completely; at that early time in a person's life there is a possibility of karma being changed. Such events—that seem to have their reason for being in concerns beyond this present life—happen in order that we may learn certain lessons, not as punishment, and there are many ways to learn. However, there are also many mysteries to life that we cannot explain.

Individual Responsibility and Its Consequences

The commonality of the inner self, the center of consciousness in each of us, links us to one another. From the energetic point of view, all of us are both constantly sending to, and receiving from, the world around us. We are continually being influenced and influencing others throughout our lives by these energetic patterns of thought and feeling. Nevertheless, we are personally responsible for how we react to these influences. Will we get swept away by them, or will we be able to remain centered enough to discriminate among the influences that bombard us daily? The choice is, and must be, individual.

It is within the patterns that we weave in our lifetimes that we create the ground or basis for the working out of karma. Many people hold a limited view of karma. They think that if I hit you, you would hit me back. That is simplistic; the concept of karma is truly more profound and far-reaching. Karma is not made up only of physical reactions; it reaches deeply into all levels of consciousness. Our interactions and activities at the different levels of consciousness become the root sources and energetic ingredients of karmic forces. They direct how the natural laws of karma and rebirth are manifested within and around us by the circumstances of life.

Karma is a spiritual law of action and the responsibility for that action. It affects our relationships with people and our environment and also how we relate to the future. We are each responsible for the way we feel and think—whether we are consciously aware of our thoughts and feelings or not—for they motivate our actions and, in turn, affect others. Our deeply held feelings, thoughts, and actions have a tremendous effect, usually through our memory of them. They are what karmically bind us, be they positive feelings such as love and friendship, or negative ones of anger, hate, or resentment.

Some of the most challenging events we face in life are brought about by our relationships. They can be the source of our greatest happiness and our deepest pains. We become bonded to the people we love, but we are also bound by those we hate or dislike. Even though our dislikes may be very reasonable in our own minds, they attach and bind us. We repeatedly think of people we strongly dislike, or those who have done us great harm, even if we are not consciously aware of it. The end result is that our thoughts keep us linked to those people.

Karma must also be thought of in the larger sense, not only in terms of the individual. We are all linked, consciously or unconsciously, to the planet and to the various groups with whom we associate. Individuals not only have personal karma; they are also connected simultaneously to the karmic patterns of the groups and countries, or regions, to which they belong, as well as to the karmic patterns of Nature and the Earth. From this perspective, what we do to the planet and how we relate to its inhabitants both have karmic consequences and affect our future as individuals.

Each country and its inhabitants make up the collective spirit of that particular area of the planet. The collective thoughts and feelings of the inhabitants of a country create the pattern of karma for that country. As an example, let us consider two countries that are at war with one another. The deaths, bloodshed, and suffering affect not only the individuals involved, but also the collective consciousness and karma of the two countries.

The collective spirit can also be a very positive force. Today there is a great spirit vigorously moving across the world, especially among young people, that stimulates interest and commitment to the concepts of ecology and environmental conservation. It means that individuals are accepting responsibility for their interactions and relationships to all of Nature and, in a sense, are becoming caretakers of Earth's karma.

The Complex Concept of Karma

I have believed in karma and reincarnation since I was a very small child. I was born in Java, in what was then the Dutch East Indies, and was brought up on the ideas of Hinduism, Buddhism, and Christianity, while being raised in a Muslim country. One of the most famous Buddhist monuments is located in Java, a land with an endless amount of Hindu temples and a population that is predominantly Muslim. Very early in life, I was involved in discussions about karma and reincarnation, and these ideas became part of my belief system and experiences. We do not realize it here in America, but more than half of the world's population is made up of Buddhists and Hindus who believe in these concepts.

In the Hindu system of Patanjali, three kinds of karma are distinguished: first, the karma of the past that bears fruit in this lifetime; secondly, the karma from the past that does not bear fruit in this lifetime but will in some future lifetime; and thirdly, the karma one is currently making, which will bear fruit in the future.

To try to explain the Buddhist concept of karma and reincarnation, a story is told about Gautama Buddha, the spiritual teacher. The Buddha is depicted as a being of great compassion and understanding. A small boy came to visit the Buddha, and Buddha talked to him in a few choice words, teaching him a few basic tenets of Buddhist wisdom. The Buddha shared with him the successes he would have in a future life. However, the Buddha, with his omniscience, also knew that the boy would be murdered soon after leaving his presence but did not tell him.

Hearing this story, many of us would say that the Buddha should have warned the small boy. However, the Buddha's compassion came from a deeper level. Totally understanding the concept of cause and effect, the Buddha felt that it was more compassionate to let the boy go through his karmic pain and suffering. The painful death experience may have been a necessary step in the child's karmic destiny, the paying of a karmic debt that may have left him free to grow and flourish in his next incarnation. And the Buddha imparted to the boy some of the fundamental principles of his teachings so that he would die with them fresh in his mind, making those thoughts first and foremost in the child's beliefs in his next life.

To many people the actions of the Buddha may have seemed cruel, but the Buddha was not looking at the boy from the point of view of one life; his compassion and vision were in terms of the boy's inner self or soul. The story is strange from a Western Christian point of view, but it is a worthwhile one if a person is trying to gain an understanding of the Eastern concept of karma and reincarnation. Everybody might not like the implication of the story, but many times life is exactly like that. Our lessons may seem hard, but they may be just what we need to truly grow in wisdom and understanding. The Buddha, through his own pain and sufferings, had awakened to true insight into the nature of suffering. The Buddha was convinced of the absolute justice of his compassion toward the boy, and through the story we can see that karma and reincarnation are really two aspects of one interwoven concept of universal justice.

There is a positive connection between accepting a spiritual path and the acceleration or removal of karma. An example may explain this. A person well known to us was stricken by polio at about the age of two, and was severely disabled and in severe pain thereafter. I have known her for twenty-five years, and I have never met anyone like her. She has been in pain her whole life, is unable to walk anymore, and is confined to a wheelchair. Yet she has maintained her cheerful and pleasant demeanor through all her physical hardships.

Even with her physical difficulties, she has learned to paint very professionally and earns her living that way, even though the act of painting is painful in itself. She has been in and out of hospitals for years and has had countless operations. What is so miraculous about her is that she strongly feels that she can make a contribution to life and to others. She feels that by being cheerful, in spite of the pain, she can be of service to others facing similar problems.

The doctors of several hospitals have used her to help patients who are concerned about a pending operation or therapy and are depressed or fearful about their future post-hospitalization. She has not only learned to accept her physically painful destiny, but also she feels that she has the strength and fortitude to help others. To me that is truly the spiritual way of living out a difficult destiny. She has learned the spiritual ideal of unselfishness and has become a living example for others. To me, she is someone who has truly obliterated and transformed a great deal of negative karma from her being, by thinking of others before herself.

I believe that many of us misunderstand the concept of time as it relates to karma. We are constantly measuring events in our lives in relation to the number of years it takes to complete a particular task. Time does have a relationship to experience, of course. However, we need to recognize that when we have a relationship with others, or are facing a situation, we are working out our karma, and whether it takes eight years or ten years does not matter in itself. It is not the length of time that is important, but what we do with that time. It is part of the Western concept of civilization that things that take a long time must be valid. To me, it is the amount of deeply felt interaction that is truly significant. Remembering a short but happy time in one's life can be more crucial than remembering long periods of difficulty and strife.

Another true story elucidates this point. When I was working with the healer Oskar Estebany in a series of healing sessions at Pumpkin

Hollow Farm, we treated a young boy who was a hemophiliac. He was brought by his father, a Greek Orthodox priest, and his mother, who physically assisted and monitored the boy in just about every act of daily living.

The boy had not been able to walk, and had never mixed with children of his own age. Mr. Estebany and I gave him healing treatments, and on the second day he was able to walk. I asked his parents' permission to let him leave their side and sit at a table with the other children. I had warned the other children beforehand to be very gentle with him. We had a dog at the Farm, which made me a bit apprehensive with the child being so frail. It turned out that the boy was ecstatic about the dog and wanted to play with him constantly. He had never played with a dog before and seemed so happy and joyous.

I personally felt a bit worried because this child—who had not walked in years, whose health was so precarious—was now running around and playing with the dog. I wanted to tell him to stop playing so much, but I felt a pang of conscience, being aware that he seemed so happy. Finally, on the last day of the sessions, his legs began to tire a great deal, and he had to curtail his activities. Nevertheless he continued to be happy when the dog sat by his side. He went home, and I am not sure whether or not he was able to walk again. But I have often thought that even if he died, he had a very happy memory. The happiness of being able to be part of the group and not be viewed as a sick child, I am sure, meant a great deal to him. It was not the amount of time he had at Pumpkin Hollow as much as the intensity of his feelings that made his sessions so beneficial. His disease may have been his karma or destiny, but during that short time he was happy, and important changes occurred in the way he regarded himself.

Changing the Course of Karma

We are living in a universe that is eternally changing. From the cells of our bodies to the galaxies in the universe, everything is in continuous movement and change. Change is one of the basic rhythms of Nature, affecting us both outwardly and inwardly. Yet we are more frightened of change than anything else. We get attached to certain ways of thinking, feeling, and acting that can bind us to habitual and ritualistic patterns of behavior.

We are all born with many potentials but most people put only a small part of their latent potentials into active use. Some people grow very little over a lifetime, and their lives often consist of dealing with one frustration after another. These people have not used their given potentials nor have they really learned anything of significance to their inner growth, so they are destined to experience the same difficulties again in some other incarnation. I would say, however, that the average person does learn a few things in a lifetime, and the essence of that learning is absorbed into the inner self.

We must learn not to be fatalistic in our conception of karma. Karma is a universal law of cause and effect, but we are also constantly putting into effect new causes by what we do, feel, and think. At times we can change the course of our karma by our decisions and choices. There are times in our lives when we are given a choice to react one way or another. Tremendous changes can occur in our lives if we have the desire to alter the present pattern of daily living, and then do the hard work to make these changes a reality. If we can originate our decision to change from an aspect of the inner self—as may occur during meditation—our decision can then penetrate into and through our feelings and thoughts and set the stage for acts of transformation.

We can alter our patterns by learning new ways of relating to people and life's situations. Even when we feel that we are too old or feel that life is changing too fast around us, we can still learn new ways and grow. We must try to recognize those aspects of ourselves that are bound by destiny, and likewise understand those that are not. From my point of view, our destiny or karma is limited to big events in life, while the ability to change our thinking and actions gives us the freedom of the human spirit. It is in the realization of the latter that we have the ability to change and grow, and thereby alter our karmic patterns to some degree.

I do not believe that every pattern of life can be changed; some are part of our destiny. An example of that is the boy with hemophilia; to me that was part of his destiny. It is our attitude that is important. Certain people I have known have learned to accept and live with their limitations, not with a sense of helplessness, but with an affirmative sense of acknowledgment. Others feel a sense of helplessness with their difficulties in life and see no prospect for the future, except suffering.

I think that life is, to some extent, a testing ground for the inner self, and often the testing concerns the relationships we have with one another. Let me give an illustration. When I first came to the United States, I came to visit with a Latin American family. From my own perspective, I felt that there was a very strong link from the past among the family members. I found out what it was when they told me the following story.

When the family was in Latin America, they had two sons. Everybody worshipped the younger brother, who was an unusually beautiful child. One day both boys climbed a tree. All of a sudden the branch broke and the boy whom everyone worshipped was killed instantly, while the other boy survived. The guilt the older boy felt for being part of that disaster was intensified, because for two or three days he could hear people saying "Why didn't *he* die?" As time passed, the situation was never resolved, setting up unspecified but rigid barriers between the surviving boy and the other family members.

The family asked for my counsel. I suggested that rather than seeing what had happened only as a terrible thing, they needed to recognize that it made them aware that it had been a great privilege for them all to have four or five happy years with the younger son. They were all uplifted by that. Then I pointed out that they needed to all draw together in the love they shared and accept the opportunity they had to support the older boy who also had been traumatized. It sounds strange, but, upon the realization of this, they turned toward one another for the first time in years and the relations that had been so painful to them for so long were mended.

I think that we have to accept that there will be events in our lives that cannot be explained. Consider all those years during which resentment had overwhelmed the loving support they should have given the older boy. They finally were able to overcome that attitude, and it changed the outlook of all concerned. Like them, we also have prejudices that have influenced our lives significantly, even though they might not have been based on the truth of a situation. Those are the things each of us can alter; conscious reflection can change karma.

Besides helping ourselves, to a certain extent we can also help others caught in the mesh of negative circumstances. These days there is a great deal of fear about the disease, AIDS, which is prevalent in the world. When many millions of people hold the same thought, it becomes a world picture or thought form. At home and at work, I am sure that many of you have mentally picked up unexpressed feelings of anger, depression, or fear in a person or people around you. Most people do not realize that they are unconsciously receiving and responding to the AIDS epidemic with fear and a sense of panic, often without good reason. These frightening emotions do not always originate within ourselves but often are acquired from the atmosphere of general thoughts that continually float through our momentary awareness.

Those who are able to practice Therapeutic Touch can make a significant contribution to persons caught in such anxieties. TT therapists are convinced within themselves, through their practice, that the energy of thoughts and feelings can be projected to someone else for therapeutic purposes. They realize that nonverbal communication is a reality, and not just mere fantasy.

In many cases I feel this type of communication is more powerful than talking. Let us take the example of being around someone who has experienced a tragedy. We may feel tongue-tied and unsure of the appropriate thing to say. It is silly to say, "I'm sorry," isn't it? At those times probably holding the person in our mind's eye and projecting thoughts of peace to them can convey the depth of our thought more appropriately than saying words that have no meaning.

Let us look at how patients with AIDS feel about the disease. This type of understanding actually applies to all of us and to all sorts of crises. Many patients with AIDS are hungry for human compassion but the atmosphere of fear that has been built up around the disease unfortunately stops many people from expressing the compassion that is needed. If we have an irrational fear, it is communicated to others. The patient is able to sense our discomfort even if it is nonverbal. The patient with AIDS faced with the prognosis of death becomes enveloped with feelings of fear and, likewise, feels a tremendous amount of anger and resentment. If we want to help these people, we—particularly those in the health fields—must look at our own resentments and fears and recognize that we may be harboring emotions that can be contagious to those who are vulnerable.

Death aɔ Tranɔition

The subject of death is a difficult one. I believe that a few things in our life are predestined; death and the moment of death fit into this category. Although death has some general characteristics, it can be a profoundly difficult personal experience for the individual. In our present civilization, death has become a difficult stage in the evolutionary process of consciousness, invoking in many a sense of fear. In American medicine, "Death" is the ultimate enemy to be overcome. Nurses and doctors who work in hospitals have been taught that they must do everything they can to combat it.

In other cultures this subject is looked upon differently. Cultures and beliefs that have a strong tie with Nature and the land are often open to believing in life after death. I can think of the religious beliefs of the Native Americans as a typical example. In ancient cultures, where death was accepted as part of the cycles, this fear was less pronounced. In countries such as India, where the major religious beliefs include ideas such as reincarnation and life after death, the country has a different atmosphere. By "atmosphere" I mean that the people have a greater acceptance of dealing with the vicissitudes of life, understanding that life is made up of cycles and stages of growth. They accept this lifetime as part of a larger cycle.

Many people believe that when we pass over, something of who we were, our consciousness, continues to live on. From my point of view, we *are* a consciousness inhabiting a physical body. When we think of someone, we often think of how he last looked; we rarely think of him as a being of consciousness. Humanity is strange in this respect. We overlook the fact that after many years the physical appearance of those around us has changed, but the part we love is still there and alive to us. The consciousness of a person contains the sum total of their emotional and mental qualities at their moment of death. The physical body becomes a lifeless shell, while the consciousness lives on. This consciousness has various stages and processes in its further development.

As I mentioned, in the United States, more so than in other countries, we think of death as the most terrible thing that can happen to a person, whereas in other countries it is taken for granted that each of us will die at some point in the future. Let us remember one thing: there is nothing living that does not die. It is a law of the universe. I think it is important to acknowledge this, particularly for those in the health professions. When a person dies is not in the hands of the TT therapist. In many circumstances the therapist may help a great deal, but I also think it is necessary to accept that the help you can give may be limited. When you are involved with or near a dying patient, whether you do TT or not, you can quietly say to them—aloud or within your mind— "Be peaceful. . . I am glad you can go." You might be the only one in the entire hospital who would think to say that. In this way, you could help make that person's passing a calm and peaceful event.

A person in the process of dying has part of his consciousness in the other world already, and if you can say, "Go in peace and I am happy for you," you alone, out of all the persons relating to him, can have a peaceful effect on that patient. You would be unique, because most others would say, "How terrible," and do little more. However, in so many cases, death can be a wonderful release after a time of intense pain, prolonged illness, or agonizing fear. If you can accept that peacefully, it will have a quieting effect on the patient. In the long run, a peaceful death of a loved one also has a calming effect on their family.

There is no way wishing a person peace could harm a person and— even though you cannot know for sure what happens when a person dies—there is the chance that you may actually do some good, whatever the destiny of the patient may be. For myself, I would take that slim chance and try it. I would give it my best effort, and try to be helpful in a situation most people in our culture think of only in negative terms. What I would like you to feel—if you find yourself in such circumstance—is that you can help, but you are not responsible for the destiny of that patient.

My personal point of view is that it is the inner self that is the focus for the cycles of reincarnation. This gives a perspective to my healing interactions with, for instance, the many people with AIDS whom I have tried to help in the past but who died. We were able to present an alternate view to them—that it is the consciousness that survives. It made it easier for them to accept their own dying, because they had a perspective from which to perceive the transition. From the point of view of the healer, one should not feel that she has failed, but that sharing this view has made it easier for those who are dying. If one accepts that the consciousness survives, the link to the person who has passed on continues. One can help that person by sending thoughts of love, and that makes the transition easier, too.

After the moment of death, there is a transition. This transitory period is when we leave the physical Earth and its concerns behind, and awaken to a new life on the other side. The person who has passed on must deal with the grief of those they left behind. The grieving person feels a sense of loss, a profound separation, often believing they will not see their friend or loved one again. At funerals waves of grieving emotions are projected outward; these feelings are picked up by the person who has passed on at the time when he is just beginning to cope with his new surroundings. He is trying to acclimatize himself to the newness of his present existence while still feeling the strong ties with those left behind, especially in the first week or so after transition.

If someone close to us has passed over, it is natural to feel a sense of loss or grief. If we wish to maintain a spiritual approach to this situation, we must ask ourselves: how can I help the person who has passed on? At this crucial period it would be most beneficial for ourselves and our loved one to try to get beyond our personal feelings of grief, and send thoughts of peace and love. Sending thoughts of love at this time can greatly help both parties. The bonds of love will be strengthened, and our connecting links to one another can deepen, transcending both earthly time and space. By sacrificing our personal feelings of grief, we strengthen our ability to go out to others in need and learn a true lesson of compassion. We still would have a feeling of separation underneath; that is normal, but it would not be our primary focus. Our wanting to selflessly help another would be foremost in our consciousness. Dealing with death in this manner makes the transition easier for all concerned.

Our overall experience after transition is based on how we dealt with life on this side. If we have been unable to deal with old habits in this life, those prejudices follow us into the next phase; if we had a limited worldview in this life, we carry the essence of that belief system into the next realm of consciousness.

We each have different personalities and see things from individual perspectives. Because our reactions to things are different, our experiences with death are also different. People who have studied about life after death seem more open, even excited about what the after-life world will be like. If someone has passed over and keeps in contact with one who is living here on Earth, the person on the other side may get an intimation about when the earthly life of their friend is about to end. Even the person with little interest in understanding death will find those they have known and loved waiting for them at their death, waiting to help them on their journey.

There are many recorded testimonies at the Society of Psychical Research, both in London and New York City, about people in the process of dying who see, and sometimes can describe, people from the other side who gather around their deathbed. At the time of death, the recognition of a visit from a dead relative or friend can be a profound experience. It can awaken a sense of confidence within us and relieve our apprehension for the new life we are about to embark upon. What if someone does not have any close ones? A compassionate stranger would act as guide for someone with no close relatives or friends.

Today many more people are aware of and open to discussions about life after death. Recent polls have shown that a majority of contemporary Americans now believe in the concept of the continuation of life after death. However, the majority of people do not perceive things from a spiritual perspective. They live life, let us say, half asleep, and death comes to them as a rude awakening. Life on the other side is a totally different world with totally different dimensions. It is very hard to describe that realm to people who are rooted in this three-dimensional, physical Earth. To truly understand that other world takes a tremendous widening of perception.

The Stages Between Death and Rebirth

From my point of view, the experience of death, the transition phases, and reincarnation are common experiences for us all, with some degree of difference for each individual. It is difficult to describe the stages between death and rebirth, so I will try to present these concepts in as simple and clear as way as possible, without relying on long and difficult foreign terminology.

Immediately after death there is still a type of continuation of the personality, as we knew it here on Earth. Over time the personality traits that make each person uniquely different slowly disappear. Habits that pertained to living in physical reality and attachments to the physical body slowly retreat into the background and fade away. Our true individuality—the talents we use and express in a lifetime—is absorbed into the inner self, a type of storehouse of energies from many levels of our consciousness. It absorbs and integrates all of what has been understood and learned in a lifetime—that is, not learning in an intellectual sense, but as true wisdom. This sum total or essence of our experiences becomes part of our inner self.

The astral world or emotional field, where we reside after our earthly life, eventually dies out too. The inner self is then immersed in a level of consciousness where the personality has been shed, and it achieves a sense of unity with the highest level of consciousness a human being is capable of attaining. It is in the nature of a reunion, in fact. This unified period, for however long it lasts, comes to an end when karmic forces reawaken us to another earthly incarnation. Ancient traditions tell us that whatever we have done to other people, rightly or wrongly, has been recorded in our individual karmic records, a very complex concept to understand. With our rebirth comes a clearing of our memory of the particulars of our previous existence, but the essence of the things we learned from our previous lifetime still exists deep in our consciousness.

It is almost impossible to explain the sense of timelessness of the inner self, even though it is a very important philosophical question. Nevertheless, one must say that eventually it becomes time for the inner self to reincarnate in a new personality. From past incarnations many links have been forged with different people and groups. In one lifetime it is probably impossible to reconnect with all the linkages we have made over time, so each lifetime we are given certain tasks to perform and a chance to reconnect with those who have also reincarnated at that time and may have similar interests. Some of the people we meet in a lifetime are those with whom we have previously bonded, either positively or negatively. In this present life we are given a new opportunity to choose how we will relate to the people with whom we had formerly bonded. Will we fall into the same types of patterns with them, or will we forge new and positive interactions? All the forces and patterns we have set into action in previous times will have the opportunity to be worked through during our lifetimes. It is, in some respects, very like a complicated computer system in which all facets of a lifetime's destiny—its lessons, relationships, and time sequences—are figured out in broad strokes.

Some people are more enlightened than others. They have experienced a great deal over many incarnations and, therefore, are more attuned to their inner self and are, in turn, of greater service to others. They have learned to put others above their personal needs and desires. People like the Dalai Lama and Mother Theresa come to mind. They have uniquely developed themselves, and react in life with a small amount of personal attachment; they are able to love in a non-attached, compassionate way. Service to the world and humanity is their key concern.

Communication with the Other Side

In the world of life after death, the common experiences of transportation and communication occur very differently, and people who have passed on learn how to experience both of these in new ways. In this world we are used to talking to each other verbally; on the other side extrasensory perceptions are common experiences. There, we do not have to open our mouths to talk; we mentally visualize the sentences and questions we wish to express. Others can mentally pick up and understand the content of our thoughts and feelings. Vocal cords, as such, do not really exist there. Language is used, but it is through thought communication, in lieu of verbal interaction, that this is accomplished.

It is not easy for people on the other side to communicate with us. The best and easiest way is for them to try to impress thoughts and ideas into our minds. Those on the other side, because they have learned to communicate by ESP, concurrently learn the ability to forcibly project their thoughts. This thought projection makes it easier for them to communicate with us, than we with them, while we are alive. Being used to talking and to language, we are not as proficient in forceful thought projection. Sometimes communication from them to us occurs during our sleep, while we are dreaming.

Some people think they get communications through psychic experiences, such as automatic writing or thought channeling. It is not usually people who are educated who get these messages. Some of the printed stuff I get is tripe. I think that if there were people on the other side who were trying to help, they would not say such ordinary things. However, there are also some valid communications. That would be a fair way of putting it.

Our unconscious is vastly more aware than our conscious minds. In these experiences we may not be actually communicating with a departed friend or relative, but instead may be tapping into some level of our own unconscious. Not many people consider this as a possible explanation for their experiences. All of us here live busy lives, dealing with our occupations and our many relationships; people on the other side are also busy with their lives. Those who have passed on are in the process of learning, living apart from us. They do not have the time to keep a twenty-four hour vigilant watch over us, nor, therefore, are they in constant communication with us. In many instances, those who think they are being directly helped by someone on the other side are unconsciously picking up insight, not from angels or people who are dead, but from the universal healing field itself.

When you are grieving for a person on the other side, it is because of your personal relationship with him or her. You feel bereft of your communications with them. What I suggest is that you can always send love to the person who has passed over. The relatives who take me up on that suggestion, whether they are adults or children, have told me later how strengthening and satisfying it was to send a deep feeling like love and to know that that love is returned even though the person who passed over is in another place. Right after the death, I think it is important to really concentrate and especially think of your love toward that person. Then you will be really helping and not absorbed in suffering over someone you think is lost to you. You are going out to the inner self of the other person, and you endow it with true love, which is the love between the two inner selves. Of course you will miss them, but the important thing is to accept that the affection is still there, even if the physical contact is not.

Sending beneficial thoughts is no guarantee of attracting another person to us, but sending them can be beneficial nevertheless. How can we know when a person who has passed on is with us? How can we discriminate between a true communication and wishful thinking? It is hard to know for certain. We have to be truthful with ourselves in these matters and not just believe what we want to believe. Sometimes direct communication comes to us as a warning or a clarification of which way to turn in life. But then again, it is hard to discern if this help has originated from a true act of communication or from a spark of intuition from our inner self. We must judge these things with wisdom, not impulse.

When we think of someone, we form an image of that person fixed in time. In human relationships it is not always easy to accept the world of change. Many of us like to keep a fixed image of those around us. However, in reality, people go through changes after death as well as in life. Some people make rapid changes; others never seem to significantly change at all. However, change and growth are different than we experience in this life. The conditions are different—without the trials and tribulations of life that are inherent in the physical world. Here we are in constant action and interaction with the thoughts and feelings of others. Life on Earth is difficult, birth is difficult; we live in a world of challenges. However, through facing those challenges, we have the opportunity to grow beyond our present state of being. We are born on Earth for just that purpose—to grow, to change, to learn.

On the other side we are not tested in the same way so we are able to stand back and view what we learned. A person who has crossed over does not necessarily change his or her temperament, but the perspective on life changes. We realize how much we were bothered by details in our earthly life. Another shift in our orientation is the concept of time. Very quickly after passing on, we experience this shift in time awareness. We no longer need to live by the clock, nor do we. These changes do alter the individual.

When we are meditating or trying to communicate we must realize that those who have passed on are not the same as when we last saw them. From their new, broader perspective they are able to better understand and comprehend us. We, too, can learn to see from this more expansive perspective while still here on Earth. Exploring philosophical and spiritual ideas can help us in this direction.

THE NATURE OF THERAPEUTIC TOUCH

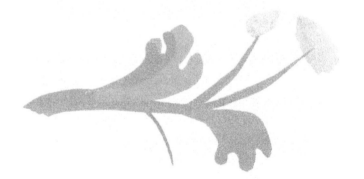

Introductory Comments

After making conscious contact with the inner self, the critical second step in the Therapeutic Touch process is the assessment. While maintaining a state of sustained centering, the TT therapist uses her activated hand chakras to explore the healee's vital-energy field of consciousness, seeking out areas of imbalance and fluctuations in intensity, rhythm, and flow. These indicants of imbalance will act as clues to the healee's state of illness. This is a learned—rather than a natural—skill, which has proven to have a high degree of reliability. It may be done by a single TT therapist, in a one-on-one relationship with a healee, or it can be done by two therapists working together on a healee. The latter method is usually done by beginners of the TT technique, so that each therapist can supplement the other's expertise; however, it also is performed in this manner by therapists who are more mature in TT practice when they are pooling their skills in behalf of a patient with very difficult or obscure problems.

The nature of the assessment is very personal, as the TT therapist explores the healee's vital-energy fields. In addition to physical symptoms, the TT therapist may pick up on the healee's emotions or thoughts because all of the healee's other subtle energy fields interpenetrate the vital-energy field. To a certain degree the healee is aware of this and, therefore, may feel open and vulnerable. Since this attitude might interfere with the therapist-healee relationship, the therapist tries to maintain an air of objectivity and be non-intrusive in her techniques, nevertheless maintaining a gentle, supportive manner, even engaging the healee in light conversation.

The very nature of the TT assessment also makes it highly subjective. Consequently, aspects of the manner in which one does the assessment are very individual. Because the assessment is based on inner experiences, TT therapists feel very free to subject their findings to peer review or to work together with a second therapist. At the same time, the therapist slowly gains a high degree of confidence in her findings as she increasingly permits the inner self to enter her daily activities and, through experience, begins to understand the familiar nature of that inner self.

Dora always advocated starting the assessment by first placing one's hands at the back of the neck, between the healee's shoulders, because she perceived that it served to relax the individual and to open him to healing energy flow. The area is well chosen, from both the Western scientific and the Eastern yogic point of view. The site she suggests overlies the brachial plexus, which feeds neural energy and blood supply from the base of the neck out to the tips of the individual's arms. It is also the place where therapists (of modalities other than Therapeutic Touch) say that ". . . the body carries stress."

I have described the Eastern view in broad terms elsewhere (Krieger, 1997), based upon an English translation of one of the ancient Hindu texts called the Upanishads. After describing the entrance of the major pranic flow through the vital-energy field overlying the spleen, and the course the pranic flows take to vitalize the major organs and tissues of the body, the text of the Upanishad then continues: ". . . When this process is completed, these units (subsystems) of prana flow and meet in the person's vital-energy field in the region between the two shoulder blades, at the confluence of the brachial plexus. They then stream down the nonphysical vital-energy complement of the person's arms to what is known as 'the knot' (*granthi* in Sanskrit) of the wrists. At the site of the knot, the pranic streams are reconstituted to their original five subsystems, and the subsystems of the prana exit, each subset through one of the five fingers."

As I noted, the TT assessment is a learned process, and one becomes better at it with experience. In effect, it is a kind of sensitivity training, as one becomes more aware of the nuances of the vital-energy flow, and possibly becomes increasingly appreciative of the deeper psychodynamic flows over time as well. In the TT assessment one becomes aware of changes or irregularities in rhythm, flow, or intensity, or in patterns of subtle energy systems that hold personal meaning for the therapist. Very often—in a manner that is difficult to describe or even to understand oneself—the bits of information that the TT therapist picks up in the healee's subtle energy fields seem to come together or to synthesize deep within her intelligence, her personal place of informed knowing. In a measureless moment the therapist has a clear visualization of the healee's problem and sometimes even gains insight into the original cause of that problem.

In the next phase of the TT process the therapist—now in possession of information about what is wrong with the healee in terms of his energy systems—devises a plan of action to restore balance to the healee's vital-energy field and perhaps also his psychodynamic field. She then goes on to carry out the plan she had conceived by using various TT techniques where they are needed. Most of the actual healing takes place during this rebalancing phase. However, time is often very different during the healing experience; in tick-tock time, healing may continue to take place after the healing session. To conclude the TT session, the therapist will then do a reassessment of the healee to determine whether the necessary rebalancing actually has occurred, and to decide whether additional TT healing is required, or whether referral to some other healing modality may be of help to the healee.

Not all patients respond fully to the Therapeutic Touch process. However, more than thirty years of clinical experience with Therapeutic Touch has taught us that the appropriate question to ask is: "What physiological and psychological systems are most sensitive to the Therapeutic Touch process?" We have found that prime among them are dysfunctions of the autonomic nervous system, which is to say, psychosomatic illnesses. Very close behind them are problems of the genitourinary system and of the lymphatic system. Beyond that, there is significant response from the musculoskeletal system.

However, if one attempts to push this body system model further, some oddities appear. For instance, in reference to the endocrine system, some bias is noted in that TT seems to have better results with females than with males. Among the females, TT works best with problems of the reproductive system. Also, for both genders, we have not had significant success with problems of the pituitary glands, although the thyroid glands and the adrenals are both highly responsive.

We also have had impressive results in our work with catatonic and also with bipolar patients; however, we have not had significant results with schizophrenic patients, except in very selective cases.

In regard to the general public, in cases where the patient displays considerable hostility to the therapist without apparent cause, or if the patient is in denial about his illness, we find that our success rate goes down to the point where we may have to refer such patients to therapists in other modalities.

In terms of general results, TT has the highest reliability in: eliciting a full relaxation response within the first two to four minutes of the TT session; in significantly reducing or bringing about a full remission of painful symptoms; and in stimulating a decided acceleration of the healing process. Lastly, if we discard the body systems model, then there have been several notable successes when TT is used to help people through their final transition in a peaceful manner, regardless of the cause of their dying. This has led to wide acceptance of Therapeutic Touch in hospices in many countries and by people of diverse cultures or divergent belief systems.

This is a vast array of effects, and we understand how a person might wonder how one healing modality can affect such a broad spectrum of results. The only answer I ever have felt satisfied with, when I've asked such questions of myself, has come from the recognition that in Therapeutic Touch we are consciously working to integrate the dynamics of our inner selves into our practice to help or to heal others. I keep in mind that it was Abraham Maslow who pointed out that as a people we are still evolving toward a fully human state. I believe that in working consciously to integrate the inner self into our daily activities, we have an opportunity to achieve an evolutionary leap, given the generally accepted model of ego-driven personality most people adhere to at this time in our history. However, it would be arrogant in the extreme to presume that our current general state of inner evolution is capable of understanding the fullness of that actualized state of consciousness to which all beings aspire. So the question of how a simple inner work such as Therapeutic Touch can do so much for so many probably will have to remain unanswered until we ourselves grow more completely into our full stature as integrated human beings.

Recognizing our shortcomings, in this section Dora discusses several human problems in relationships with others or in self-understanding that might stand in the way of the TT therapist's ability to help or to heal those in need, or that might curtail a healee's ability to open himself fully to healing opportunities. In presenting her concept of personal growth, she emphasizes the need for the person who aspires to healing others to first order her own life. This advice is not only for one's own sake, but also for the healee's welfare, for when the TT therapist projects healing energies, she is also projecting to the healee whatever energetic flows are dominant within her fields at that time. For instance, a TT therapist who feels anxious while trying to heal someone is caught up in a disquieted, jittery, restless flow. As a result, the energy patterns that are being projected to the healee are actually loaded with the therapist's anxiety. They can play themselves out in the healee as worry and tension about his own concerns. They can also act to tinge his feelings with mistrust of the healer, because of the "bad vibes" he is picking up.

However, we do not have to be conditioned by our emotions; we harbor the potential to realign them and often thereby to transform our lives. In yearning to help or to heal those in need, we can move beyond our self-made restrictions of personality as our vital-energy and psychodynamic fields become more pliant and sensitive in reaching out to others. The pursuit of Therapeutic Touch as a healing way fosters the discipline of controlling impulses and negative emotions, for they are an expression of one's psychodynamic field, the medium through which the inner self can tangibly declare itself in acts of daily living. For instance, if a therapist becomes confused about the symptoms a healee displays during the practice of TT, she can take refuge by quieting herself through sustained centering, confidently reaching within herself for the sense of deep peace and stillness that is a metaphor for her link with the inner self, and free up the pathways to intuitive insight. This avenue to clarity of thought can also be used in resolving perplexing problems of daily life.

In another vein, Dora presents her concept of the sensitive child. She defines the sensitive child as having a personal psychodynamic field that is easily affected by other persons' emotions, but as lacking the ability to release those high energy patterns and let them diffuse naturally. The continual build-up of charged emotions can make that person highstrung, hypersensitive, and acutely reactive to persons and to circumstances. In a TT therapist, these attributes act to vitiate one's aspirations to be a calm and peaceful medium for healing. However, a person who can accept her symptoms of intense sensitivity and learn to work constructively with them may become empathetic to others who also have been caught in the negativity of extreme sensitivity, and perhaps be able to help them to heal their high state of stress. Such an empathic act can bring insight into one's own former times of unbearable sensitivity, which adds to the pleasure and satisfaction of helping others.

Observing TT therapists for over thirty years has made me aware that many came from backgrounds of being sensitive children. They have learned to deal constructively with problems that stemmed from that condition, and how to use that sensitivity in positive ways for the benefit of others who are now as they once were. It is in this more positive pursuit—the engagement of one's inner self during the healing session to help someone overcome a disability one once had—that the full powers of transformation are exercised. One gains confidence as a former weakness or lack of control is perceived to transform into a positive power. As the self-image shifts into a more life-affirmative frame of self-reference, one realizes that a once disturbing sensitivity can become a welcome ally when joined in an effort to help others similarly distressed.

Dynamics of
Therapeutic Touch

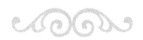

Therapeutic Touch Assessment

WE ORIGINATED THE PROCESS of assessing a patient's vital-energy field when we developed Therapeutic Touch. Mr. Estebany—the healer mentioned previously—did something similar insofar as he would put his hands on a person's body and say where he felt the illness was, but making the process simple and explicit so that it could be easily taught is one of the unique aspects of the TT method. From the beginning, we have felt that this is an important part of the healing process, and throughout the thirty years of the development of Therapeutic Touch we have devoted considerable time to studying how the assessment can be done to help those who are ill.

We recommend that you begin by standing behind the person you are healing. Put your hands on their shoulders and concentrate on relaxing them. Some people resist if they see you, but will accept your treatment if you stand where they cannot see you. When you assess a person, you are quiet within as you center. That helps you to develop the ability to be sensitive and also to forget yourself, to be wholly there for the patient's needs. This is easier to do during the assessment than during the rebalancing or healing. Then you open yourself up and your sensitivity sharpens.

You are taking in as you go outward, toward the patient. When you put your hand in their vital-energy field, you become more sensitive at your emotional level of consciousness; you expand your aura. At this point you are not trying to project or send energy; you are trying to receive information. You try to pick up—through your hands and your mind—what the problem of the patient might be. However, keep in mind that at no time are we asking you to diagnose a particular disease. What we are asking you to do is to pick up pain, fatigue, and other signs of energy imbalance. This capacity is not something that you can acquire overnight. It takes some time—maybe a month or more—to strengthen the ability to assess.

When you first start doing Therapeutic Touch you may feel a particular sensation such as heat or cold or tingling when your hands are near particular areas of the patient's body. Your individual reactions act as personal indications of pain or other symptoms. There is no one universal cue; the cues vary with the problem and with the TT therapist. No two people are alike. We all have our similarities, and we each have our uniqueness also. What you experience is *your* way of finding the problem. Another therapist may feel the cues—the heat, the cold, the tingling, and so on—differently. At the same time that you feel the sensation in your hands, something will flash in your mind. The particulars are not important. What is important is that you experience your interaction with the patient while you continue to maintain your state of centered consciousness.

Early on, some people will say they feel nothing when they put their hands over a patient, but recognition of sensation comes with practice. The reason people cannot do it initially is that their minds erase the early impressions, and all sorts of images take their place. So, when you begin, give yourself a moment or two to empty your mind as you center, and then try to pick up the impressions. It is best to go with your first impression. If you wait too long and let your mind wander, it will get a dozen ideas and you can get terribly confused.

In actual situations, there is nothing wrong in asking the patient whether the problem is located where you are picking up cues. For instance, you can ask if they feel pain in that place. If you don't ask, you will not get any verification. When you are beginning, talk softly and ask, "Am I right?" If you ask, your mind will learn to trust itself. If they say "Yes," you can then go on to do the TT rebalancing of that site and do the best you can to help them. Even if they say "No," you may ultimately be right in some way or another, but take the patient's word and go from there. You will determine the validity of your assessment as the TT session proceeds.

⟳ Models for Therapeutic ⟲
Touch Technique

I always begin by putting my hands on the back of the shoulders of the ill person to relax him, because I personally believe that only someone who is relaxed can take in the full force of healing energies. It is easy to access tension in the back of the head and neck. I also recommend standing behind the person while doing the initial stages of TT because the patient will be less aware of what you are doing as an intrusion if he does not see your face.

As I place my hands on the ill person, I am quiet, for I am taking a few moments to meditate and make the initial link with my inner self and his inner self. In this way we can make a connection at an impersonal but "high" or "deep" level. Putting the hands on the shoulders is really the crucial beginning of the healing, because in that moment the healer begins to draw upon the healing reservoir, the universal healing field.

If you are in the position of not knowing what to do for a patient who is very disturbed emotionally—perhaps you do not know the diagnosis and your own experience is limited—start, of course, by centering and feeling this peace yourself. Some people are so disturbed that it takes away from their being able to accept the full healing. If you simply send a sense of calm and peace to help a disturbed person quiet down before you actually do the healing, then he will be in a peaceful state of mind, and it will be easier for his body to absorb the healing energies. From my experience, many people will respond.

After centering, you then go on to assess. In your assessment, you are not diagnosing a disease; you are evaluating the cues you are picking up—the heat, the cold, and so on. What you can pick up very quickly is pain. You then put your hand where you feel the cue, and simultaneously you expand your emotional field and also heighten your sensitivity. Then you open yourself up by the treating or balancing of the cues. You reach out to help, and increasingly—in your sensitivity and compassion—you draw upon the universal healing field.

When you are working with a partner, it is a good idea to take a moment to center together before doing TT. For one thing, the healing energy does not begin at once; it takes a few moments to begin to flow through you. During the time you are centering and being still, this flow "catches up" with your projection and intention; from then on it flows more fully and in accord with the situation.

TT therapists in general are remarkably good in assessing pain. As I watch them during healing sessions, directing or modulating healing energies, they unconsciously and naturally have their minds concentrated on what they are doing. They particularly focus on where they have picked up pain and help to reduce it. But sometimes the basic pattern of the disease actually shows up somewhere else and they miss that connection. The energy structure of pain being sent out from the body seems to have "sharp edges," making it more distinctly marked than other energy. A disease is different, because it is on a more subtle level—actually several levels of consciousness simultaneously—and its effects are more diffuse.

While a patient's pain is one of the first things a TT therapist learns to become aware of, there are other sensitivities one can develop and deepen. I recommend that you open your mind a little further and realize that there may be other, less sharply felt, centers of disorder. See if you can go a little bit further than just assessing the pain; go on to discern the secondary pattern of the disease. Then you'll be able to send healing energies through the center of the disease as you do now. And—by paying attention to that secondary pattern—you will add intentionality to your healing effort, increasing its effectiveness considerably.

In some cases a disease process can begin before there are any symptoms. I remember a funny story in this regard. A Danish author wrote on the life of Swedenborg, and she was very skeptical about his clairvoyance. We met because she wanted to talk to me about that. In the process of our conversation I said that I thought she was developing some problem with her kidneys. She looked straight at me and said with great confidence, "I have no pain in my kidneys. I have nothing the matter with me." One week later she called to tell me that she had a virulent kidney infection, and that I had been right. We became very good friends until the end of her life.

There is a progression in the practice of Therapeutic Touch. First you become aware of the pain. Then, slowly and with experience, you become aware of the various levels of consciousness. Then over time you may develop this level of insight, having gained a great deal more confidence in the total healing process. You may pick up an indication of a disease in Therapeutic Touch, but if you are beginning, you have to learn by asking the patient until you get a sense of certainty about it. After a while it is remarkable how well Therapeutic Touch therapists are at finding the source of a problem even if it is in a different place than the pain.

Most of you can pick up the symptoms of arthritis in a patient. The pain is in the joints, of course, and you can put your hands on the top of the knee joint and pick up cues such as heat or cold. You do not feel it as pain; you feel it as these cues, whereas a person who has done Therapeutic Touch for some time could probably actually feel the pain for a few moments when she put her hands into the patient's vital-energy field. You most frequently feel the energy flow as "blocked," and describe it as lack of flow. As you begin to rebalance the area, you say you can feel an increasing flow.

You also have to learn how to reach the healing part of the patient; that is a different way of looking at sensitivity. When you look at a knee, you think of the energy as flowing down, but you also need to think of the totality of that being—that individual as related to the entirety of the energy systems outside, in the environment and universe. Then, what you try to do, in a sense, is to realign it organizationally with itself, as it would be in a normal state. As I mentioned previously, you do have to be quiet for a moment as you are treating a person, to try to get at these deeper levels of the healing interaction. I do not think you will be able to right away, but if you continue to practice, I think you will become more aware.

Relating to the Inner Self

On the basis of more than a quarter of a century of experience, research, and analysis, we believe that there is a healing power with a consciousness that helps you as you pick up the symptoms in the Therapeutic Touch assessment. The idea of a consciousness that understands the circumstances of an individual's illness is foreign to Western culture, so I am trying to search for language to adequately express it.

In Therapeutic Touch we always reach to the center of peace in ourselves for a moment before we act to heal a person. Then we are feeling the calmness within ourselves as we genuinely go out in compassion to someone who is ill. We are not just putting out our hands to assess; we are trying to reach the person at his or her deepest level.

At first, when you try to pick up what is wrong with a patient, you are reaching out to know that there is an inner self in that person, and you work from there. In doing that, you might get a sense of how you can foster the capacity of the person's inner self and his mind to work together to help him heal. His mind is hooked to the pattern of the illness, but you might get an insight into how to reach him at a deeper level than the one at which he feels the pain. Therapeutic Touch—in which you are thinking of sending healing energy—enables you to reach to a deeper level than those people who are just expressing a kindness. In your compassionate concern, you are "opening up" to your own higher levels of consciousness.

Some people who are sick are ready for a therapeutic relationship at this level of consciousness, and they receive a feeling of peace and get closer to their own inner selves during the TT interaction. At that moment there is an opportunity to reach a patient while he wants to change. The patient may see himself in a new way, and a different healing process begins. However, the patient himself must respond; you cannot impose your will. You can impose less pain, you can impose less anxiety, but that deeper part of the patient must contribute from within himself.

It takes confidence in your capacity to reach your own inner self to appreciate the depths of insights you may have about patients, and sensitivity to realize the longings they may have but not be able to express.

If you can do it, you may help them toward a different life and a different way of healing.

To illustrate this point, let me tell you of an incident that took place some years ago when I spoke at a college. Out of the blue I was introduced to a very cultivated lady I had never met before. I realized at once that she was ill and—although I do not usually do this—I invited her out to lunch on a strange hunch. As I got a sense of her, I found that she was uncomfortable, not sick in the usual sense of that word. She later told me that she had multiple sclerosis and was in some pain, that she had lost her husband, and other details of her life. In our conversation, it came out that she felt that she was useless. I could not treat her in a public restaurant, but I invited her to talk to me privately.

At that time I had an insight about what she could do to express herself, a way to take her mind beyond her immediate physical condition and work out her true gifts. I realized that—although she was depressed about her physical condition—she had innate abilities to become an artist. I knew someone who could teach her how to paint and she began to develop that talent. Interestingly, the first piece that she painted for an exhibit was black and gray. She had a mind-picture of her illness, and this was her way of getting at the pain and misery of it. After that she found that she really had a gift for painting. She became a participating member of society, and her symptoms did not bother her for very many years. She died about twenty years later, but she had a sense of fulfillment. One insight changed her whole life.

If—as with several healers I have seen—there is an instantaneous healing, the inner self plays a crucial part in the process. That is only possible, I am convinced, when it is a person's karma to be healed in this way. It may also be the karma of the healer that brought her into contact with the healee. If you keep calm, whatever the circumstances, you will be able to help that person to absorb the energy to do whatever can be done. It is important that you continue to be a vehicle, sending healing energy for the ten or fifteen minutes that you are doing TT, knowing that your destiny has given you this opportunity to compassionately help another.

Lourdes, in France, is one of the largest healing centers in the world. Thousands of people pilgrimage to Lourdes each year, some with very intense religious feelings, but very few people are healed. It is a mystery why only some people are healed, but the majority are not. A great many people are enriched by the experience, because when they pray and take part in the ceremonies they reach a larger, deeper sense of consciousness. However, the actual, physical healing is extremely rare.

We who practice Therapeutic Touch are not the greatest healers in the world. We cannot touch a person, look at him in a certain way, and effect an instantaneous cure. I have met some people in India who could do that but, I must emphasize, it is very rare. My personal feeling is that in cases of instantaneous healing, the inner selves of those who were healed knew their karma ahead of time, knew that an aspect of themselves would be able to contact that universal healing field through their religious expression, their personal belief, or other aspiration. That was their destiny, being able to meet the right people or to go to the right places where the healing would occur.

Helping to Bring Order out of Disorder

You should not be over-anxious to succeed as a healer. For you to be successful you have to be as calm as you possibly can, not letting yourself be devastated by the suffering of the healee, nor taking that agony within you. You are calling upon the universal healing field—its energies are flowing through your hands—to bring order into the gravely disordered field of the ill person. Never forget that is the purpose of Therapeutic Touch: *to bring order into a disordered field.*

When you heal, in the rebalancing, you drop all attention to the outside and focus your consciousness in your heart, and then you become aware of peace and quietness. In that stillness you get a sense of the inner self, perhaps for the first time. Although you may not think of it in that way, it also means that the inner self of the patient has to some extent become present to you. If you can reach some level of the inner self—and the degree depends on both the patient and yourself—you send that energy through your hands.

Wherever there is disease, disorder has taken over. In the TT process you want to send the patient's body enough energy to fight its own disorder. If you know where the seat of the problem is, you can think of the energy going there. The patient's body will absorb some of that energy, making a greater concentration of energy available in the diseased area. Throughout all of this you are thinking of sending peace and order. That is the key. The physical body that is ill has to be willing to accept the healing; you cannot force the issue. The consciousness of the whole body uses the energy for healing within the constraints of the person's destiny.

In Therapeutic Touch you have to deal with life and death. You need to realize that the total healing process also includes helping persons in final transition. There are some very serious diseases that are hard to cure partly because they arise out of a person's karma. TT can help to reduce the pain, but cannot eliminate the disease, except sometimes in the case of children, for they have a strong possibility of change.

The Nature of Human Relationships

I believe that relationships are not so much between personalities as between consciousnesses, the total, essential consciousnesses of the persons involved. It is from this perspective that a true picture of karmic relationships can be gained. Although what we may call to mind when we think of someone is their personality and their physical appearance when we last saw them, I think that the person's consciousness is what we basically relate to over time. Whether people change or not, we think of their personality characteristics as their total being—how they feel, how they act and interact—and certain of these characteristics relate to the essential consciousness of that person.

When we see a person after a gap of fifteen or twenty years, we may hardly recognize him or her. In my travels I see people who have grown from tiny youngsters to mature young men and women, and I frequently do not know who they are, they have changed so. I remember once I was standing on a platform waiting for a ferry and two young men came out of the crowd and hugged me. I frankly did not know them at first. It was only after a few minutes that I realized they belonged to a family who were friends, whom I had not seen for several years. Although at first I may not remember someone I have not seen in a long time, in a very few minutes I recall the person's consciousness, even though I may not remember his or her name.

In life, people change, but our affection—our going out to them in a relationship—is to the sum total of their characteristics throughout their life. We feel these levels of consciousness to some extent when the Therapeutic Touch assessment is done. I think in today's world, which is passing by so fast, if we can understand and accept this point of view, we can better fulfill our role as caregivers. Thinking of a person not only as a changing personality, but also seeking out their essential consciousness, one can bring to a relationship a totally different perspective that can be very meaningful for those involved.

When a person dies and we think of him or her, we really are thinking of that person's consciousness. If you have a sense of the continuation of consciousness, then you can better help a person who is passing on. From my point of view, the recognition has an effect, even on the other side, after that person has died.

One of the hardest things I have ever had to do concerned a world-famous pianist who had heard about me and asked me to come to see him. He had called me because his son had just committed suicide, but I did not think he knew very much about philosophical ideas. As it turned out, he liked me. When we met, I talked very simply about ideas concerning life after death and asked him to sit still with me and just feel peace toward his son. Even in that short time, quietly doing something for his son gave him relief from his grieving. The suffering caused by the death of somebody comes out of the feeling that the relationship is over. That is why I advise the sufferer to send love to the person who has died. In sending that love, one begins to realize over time that the relationship has not been cut off, but continues, even after death.

I want to suggest something similar to you, for if you can reach the quietness of your own inner self, and then surround an emotionally upset person with that deep-seated quietness, he will absorb those calming energies. From an energetic point of view, what you are trying to do is to think of the upset person's subtle energy fields as being smooth. So send out not only love, but also thoughts that are strong enough to help to smooth out the jitters—the emotional upheavals—in his energy fields. Everyone I have ever tried this with has rapidly responded to the quietness and the sense of peacefulness, which help them to quiet themselves.

Too often when someone is grieving we think we have to talk, but this is something we can do without saying a word, unobtrusively. Particularly at times when you do not know what to say, the quiet sending of emotions can be very helpful. It is as effective as anything you might say, because sometimes the person is so upset he does not listen to you. All of us have done something like this without thinking about it at some point in our lives. What I am trying to put forward here is that you can do it *consciously*. You can do it more often and you will gain a great deal more self-confidence in being able to help when words are insufficient.

Emotional Obstructions to the Healing Flow

Now one can ask, what blocks the healing energy flow? One of the things I would like to discuss is the tendency many TT therapists have of talking to the patient too much. When you do Therapeutic Touch, it is good to do whatever talking needs to be done in the first few moments of the session. After that it is better—for the purpose of a deeper communication between the patient and yourself—if you talk less. This will foster your capacity to get in touch with the inner self of the patient, with their wholeness.

Every day of our lives we are exchanging feelings with others, and sometimes we sense the sadness or difficulties of patients and others in need. Very often we go out in sympathy as we pick up some of that emotional atmosphere, and it affects us. The moment you are personally affected it reciprocally impacts how you project healing energies and you become less efficient. If you are very tired, I suggest that you do very little of the healing, because you need to have an overabundance of your own energy to do TT without drawing on your own reserves. Some of you do not have the power of concentration or the sensitivity to expand or penetrate the healee's vital-energy field; how much healing energy you can transmit depends upon that.

Another problem may arise for those of you who have a tremendous desire to succeed when you try to heal. If you see somebody very sick, you automatically want to help him. You may become terribly concerned about his condition, about whether you will be able to help, and so on. These personal emotions get in the way of being centered. It is important to realize that when you pour out enormous amounts of healing energy toward someone, you may help him to reduce his pain and anxiety for the time being. But it sometimes is not a true healing. Rather, it is the result of your sensitivity to the patient's feelings.

The trouble is that—when you are exceptionally engrossed in helping a person get well—your feelings get confused with the patient's feelings. You forget the importance of remaining absolutely calm and peaceful and centered, and that you are just the instrument of the healing process. So it is very important to remember not to get overpowered by your intense feeling of wanting to help. Too much of that kind of projection throws your own feelings into it, vitiating the natural and untainted energy flowing from the universal healing field.

If your emotions do get entangled with those of the patient, your healing will only affect the patient for a little while and will not bring permanent or deep relief. At times, being a Therapeutic Touch therapist is much harder than being an ordinary therapist and just doing your best. In Therapeutic Touch you are trying deliberately—whatever your desire or compassion is—to be calm and quiet within yourself; to stop and consider the effects of your intervention *every time* you do TT. In this quiet, you try to have a sense of unity with your inner self, which is peaceful and quiet. Only then do you think of the suffering of the patient and of your energy going out to help him in compassion. The calmness that you send with intentionality is stronger than vague sympathy. Sympathy is a very necessary faculty to us, but if you are overcome by sympathy and do not recognize that you can be an instrument for healing energy, it makes a difference.

Learning how to help people feel at peace at all levels of consciousness is one of the hardest things for TT therapists to do. In most disease processes it is not only the physical organs that are in disarray; the patient is also feeling a lot of anxiety. When the TT therapist does her assessment, she is in a sense tuning in to two levels of consciousness, the physical and the emotional. Between the pain and the anxiety, which may also be tinged by fear, a novice in Therapeutic Touch might be overwhelmed by the strong emotions.

That is why it is so important to learn to be very quiet within when something traumatic happens and people are in great pain. You have to be very calm, because healing is really a very difficult job. Instead of automatically saying, "It's horrible," and shrinking from a situation, you can help the suffering person a great deal if you can send calming thoughts. What you must keep in mind is that while the person is suffering, the inner self is beyond the level of suffering. It is aware of it, one could say, but it does not have the suffering. It is a matter of not reacting, but compassionately offering another perspective to the person. But if you get too personally involved with your patients, you can become overwhelmed and forget that what happens to the patient is ultimately not in your hands.

Another problem that TT therapists have is with recurrent anxiety. The very anxious person could attempt to heal, but she would not be doing it to the fullest extent. You can still be an instrument for healing, but you are fundamentally blocked by the anxiety. In doing Therapeutic Touch, therefore, part of you will reach the patient but you will not be as clear or effective.

Truly centering yourself is one part of the answer to this problem, but acknowledgement is another aspect of which you should be aware. If you deny your anxiety—and so many people are anxious but will not admit it—then you are denying what you are at this moment. But if you can say, "I am anxious," you make that emotional pattern available to your consciousness. Then you can center your consciousness while saying to yourself, "I am going to become quiet within." Then try to concentrate on that innermost place of stillness, and go on with the Therapeutic Touch session. In doing this you become therapeutically involved with a fresh flow of *prana*, which will help the state of anxiety to abate and your emotions to repattern.

♨ Repatterning Your Anxiety ♨

Begin by centering. By doing this, you make the decision to put the anxiety aside.

Acknowledge your anxiety.

Make a deliberate effort to do something for somebody else, such as Therapeutic Touch. The energy that you engage to work beyond your personal problem will also help to unblock you.

Some people will feel that they cannot get access to the level of consciousness needed to make the acknowledgement. Then, of course, they cannot use this method to get beyond the personal need for anxiety. If you are terribly anxious, I think it is perfectly right, absolutely logical, that you have lost this contact with yourself and cannot use your will, which is what this is all about. However, most of you have a deep desire and interest in doing Therapeutic Touch, and the genuine motivation to help someone else makes you able to do a lot of things.

I know it is very hard to be honest with yourself and say, "I am anxious." You feel it is a weakness in your character, don't you think that is true? Not many people like to acknowledge that. But if you are very anxious, you are basically thinking of yourself; part of you is locked up inside of yourself, so to speak. If you can objectively say to yourself, "I am very anxious at this moment," then part of you will be looking at yourself with awareness, enabling you to deal with it.

Like anxiety, depression also negatively impacts a person's ability to do Therapeutic Touch. As energy patterns, the two emotions have something in common because they both block a person in, thereby cutting down on the outward flow of energy. The depressed person does not want to be in a depression, but he gets surrounded by it, and it is very hard for him to get out of it until the cycle of depression is over.

When you do Therapeutic Touch, you are reaching out from being sad to help someone else. Then your energy goes outward to the periphery of the field, in the opposite direction, one might say, from the in-turned flow of the depression. Otherwise, that inward flow feeds off itself and reduces your energy level. It is at those times—when you feel closed off from the flow of everything—that you lose your sense of wholeness and feel alone. But when you make the effort to go out to help others, to heal, you can break the cycle. Once again let me emphasize: *it is you who must make the effort*; that is the dynamic.

Every day we are confronted with a range of experiences, problems, and decisions, some very difficult. That is part of living, of interacting with people and events as they pass us by, often unaware of their effect on us. None of us can stay centered twenty-four hours a day, and we succumb to negative attitudes.

When something bothers you, you get upset and send out that disturbance to others, and you do not know what to do. I suggest that you say, "My feelings are hurt, and I do not want to be that way." You can acknowledge the cause, even fleetingly, and perhaps give yourself a few moments to feel the sensation of having your feelings hurt. Then do something to have your feelings go out in another way. Your feelings have been hurt for a few minutes, true, but then you are consciously doing something about it. You are saying, "No, dwelling on that is not what I want to do; that is enough." The critical thing is not to think about your emotion as coming from outside of yourself. Recognize it for what it is and admit, "*I* am reacting in that way."

When I am angry, for instance, I accept things as they are; I acknowledge that I am reacting at that emotional level. I don't think the anger comes from outside myself. I tell myself that at the emotional level I am taking things very personally, or my feelings have been hurt, and I have responded in anger. Then I say to myself, "Hey! Here I am, angry! Let me realize that there is also within myself calm and wisdom." I think of something that symbolizes the beauty and stillness of Nature, such as a tree or a mountain or an ocean. This recalls the sense of calm and beauty to that level of my consciousness as I come back to the principle involved and say, "Why was I angry?"

If you are very angry, you may not know why you are angry, so try to be at peace for one moment; think of something else, and then come back to the problem, asking yourself, "Why was I so heated up?" This may prevent you from doing something impulsive, and perhaps hurtful, to others. For instance, if you are angry with your child, you may say cruel things to him or her, you may even harm the child. But before you lose control, perhaps you could say to yourself, "For one minute let me acknowledge that I am angry. I need to punish my child, but let me feel that quietness within for one minute." Then think of that child who has behaved very badly, and accept that. Stopping for that moment would prevent you from inflicting injury on that child, first of all. It is the strength of your emotions, the anger, that does the harm. In the moment of reflecting on your anger, you will feel your love for that child, and that will also make you more reasonable.

We often do not realize that we disturb our whole body rhythm when we are constantly worried, in despair, or highly anxious. In addition, we expend a lot of energy when we are disturbed, and we establish a pattern as we permit the disturbance to recur. That strengthened pattern can take over as a prominent characteristic of our personality, and we may project that sense of disturbance to the healee when we are in a TT session.

What can we do about that? Most people can gain a sense of quiet when they meditate. Also, through meditation, we can learn to look at ourselves more dispassionately. If we take the time to look at ourselves in this way, we can see that our dysfunctional pattern is not of our true self. You will find that if you take a few minutes two or three times each day to recapture the sense of quietness, you can eliminate these disturbed patterns and re-establish your whole-body rhythms, thereby also eliminating many of the symptoms of fatigue and other psychosomatic ailments.

You can help to break your emotional habit patterns by focusing your attention for one or one and a half minutes, on something in Nature, such as a tree—a living thing that conveys a sense of peace to you. It will increase your sensitivity to the tree as well. If you do not have a live object at hand, think of a symbol that conveys an out-going emotion, such as peace or love. This is very useful when you are surrounded by very painful expressions and get caught up in the anguish. If you can stop whatever you are doing for one minute and think of that symbol, it will provide a structure of order to your subtle energy flows and thus act to conserve your energy instead of frittering it away in often useless worry.

Having an understanding of these emotional dynamics is helpful, both to yourself and to others. It is an amazing fact that one person who is quiet, in control of her emotions, and who can think positively, can send out calming thoughts that can make an incredible difference, even in a room full of disturbed people. When we want to project a healing energy and send it to a person through Therapeutic Touch, we are unconsciously thinking of wellness or balance. That is what we are trying to project. By doing so, we add to the balance of positive energies in difficult situations.

I think we would feel differently about our doing Therapeutic Touch if we realized that we had the opportunity to help in this way. Sending out thoughts of peace can significantly affect the atmosphere. Such thought, clothed in intentionality, will go much further to help a person make positive changes in his life than is usually realized. Sometimes when a person is sick, the patterns of anger or fear he has built in a lifetime of resentment can still be in his being. When we do TT we have to deal with such patterns. If the person talks to you about it, often he will say, "I cannot help that anger, I cannot change." However, I have noticed in the different groups I have worked with that sometimes a person *can change*. If a person, however sick, can reduce his resentment or anger before he passes on, it helps him to die peacefully. Helping a person to do that is an immeasurably good thing to do.

The Patient's Role in the Healing Process

In the practice of TT there are times—no matter how much you want to help—when the patient's body will respond very little and not be able to absorb the healing energy flow. If you are quiet, and really try not to concentrate on the weaknesses of the patient, but try to reach out for his strengths, you might get a sense of how you can bring about a fuller involvement of those strengths for the benefit of the patient.

However, there are many difficulties that are not always apparent that determine whether a person will be healed. The prime factors in the patient that impact the healing flow are: his own destiny; his willingness to engage himself in the healing process, that is, to allow it to happen; and his ability to relax or to permit others to help him relax, so that the healing energies can most easily and smoothly permeate his body.

Very often what blocks the effect of healing energies is that the patient has become completely identified with his disease and it has become an intrinsic part of his consciousness. Many patients who have been ill a very long time have made a picture in their mind of their sickness, and they have begun to think of it as part of themselves. They may want to be healed, but at that mental picture-making level they have a persistent image of themselves as sick. Everybody who has pain or who has been sick for a long time is hooked to a cyclic, repeating pattern of pain. The "hook" itself has something cyclic to it, and it catches the patient unawares. Then he begins to identify with the hook. When you project healing energy, that identification acts as a barrier and prevents healing from happening. It may take more healing force than you had expected to break through that mental picture.

It is for this reason that you want to give yourself time to be sensitive at this deeper level, and send healing thoughts, but continue to keep your mind open. For healing to occur, the built-up years of identification have to be overcome. The patient himself may be completely unaware of this, and it becomes a matter of helping him to gain insight into a process that is in effect keeping him from recuperation. To get by this mindset, I think you could just tell the patient to feel relaxed and nothing more. You do not want him to think about the sickness; you do not even want him to think about getting well. It is much better if he is completely relaxed so that his body will readily absorb the healing energy you are sending. Then there is the possibility that he will change his mind about being so hooked to his sickness process.

This is why I very frequently tell my patients, "Don't think that you *are* the illness. Rather, it is important to say, 'I *have* an illness.'" In this way, one recognizes that there is always a difference between one's inner self and the body that carries the disease process. Saying: I "have," rather than I "am" an illness, is, I think, the beginning of self-healing. You will find that the patients who can do that to any extent can respond far better than those who identify with the illness.

Again, let me make the important point that the TT therapist should not get too attached to the results of the healing, for the bottom line rests with the destiny of the patient and we must accept that reality. Have the courage to recognize that if the patient does not get well, part of him does not want to, or he is restricted in some way. However, those cases are extremely rare, because invariably you can help a person to some extent.

Using Visualization to Dispel
the Mindset of Illness

After I have worked with a patient two or three times I find it useful to ask him to think of a light or a color that he likes and to visualize it streaming through his body. Focusing on this imagery will help him to dispel the picture he has made of himself as being sick and break through that mindset. To ensure his involvement in his own healing, ask: "Do you feel better?" just to get his response. If he gives an answer, it indicates that mentally he is acknowledging his involvement and is willing to be responsive to the healing process.

Even sick people can help others in various ways. The very few people I have met who were able to rise above their illness or circumstances or whatever was involved realized that they could call upon other aspects of themselves. In this way they discovered that they have a lot of reserve with which to make a contribution to life. Such people really have a lot to give to others, and they do. Those I have known who have done this die peacefully and fulfilled, and those who remember them do not think of them as a "sick person," but as their friend. I think that is a life well lived, and that is the important thing. This is why I say it is important to have the attitude of: "I *have* a sickness," "I" being one's inner self, rather than: "I *am* sick."

Therapeutic Touch and Personal Growth

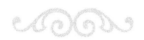

The Sensitive Child

IN GENERAL, I THINK OF HUMANITY as being divided very roughly into two kinds of personality. Everyone picks up the numerous energies of other people but one type of person naturally rejects them, expelling them from their personal field into the surrounding atmosphere. The other type of person retains these energies and is deeply affected by them. I call a person in the second group a sensitive child, one who is very sensitive and vulnerable. This is a very rough breakdown and, for the most part, people are a mixture of both types of reaction.

When small children with this kind of sensitivity are in the presence of others who are experiencing violent feelings, the energy that has been expelled by those emotions hits them. They do not understand what it is, and they often resort to crying in their bewilderment, fear, or despair. If I were angry, this kind of child would pick up some of my anger and it would remain longer in his field, influencing him, although he might not know what it was all about.

Sensitive children have a tough job because they cannot explain why they are upset when they are picking up the violence of others' feelings; they just react to the disturbance by crying or getting angry. They may scream or yell and their parent may feel that they are naughty. As these children grow, they are often difficult to handle because, to a certain extent, they will always have this sensitivity. Even when they are adults, they may suddenly come into contact with a strong emotional situation and become upset. When that happens, they do not know how to handle it. They may never fully recognize why they react to certain people in a particular way. It is a faculty they will have all their lives; however, as they grow older, they will begin to understand it better and perhaps learn how to control their reactions.

The second type of person also feels the energy sent by others. However, that energy is automatically dissipated and they are not so affected by emotional storms. Their innate ability to expel or reject the violent emotional patterns of others enables them to lead more even or balanced lives. Most people roughly conform to one of these two types, although there are admixtures of course. This basic difference between the two types may be hereditary, since the personality seems cast at birth, or there may be other constitutional factors.

These are some of the circumstances that surround the birth of the physical body and one's emotional response, and the child grows up with that. The sensitivity that people often start with when they are young is frequently misunderstood by parents or others; they feel it is temperament and not that the child cannot help picking up something. Some people who are very sure of themselves and very violent often don't think about the tremendous effect they may have upon a sensitive child. Misunderstandings often arise because of the sensitivity of the one and the strength of the emotions of the other.

So many people I have talked to remember all their lives that they were somewhat scared when they were children by the tremendous strength of what another person felt, and when they were scolded they felt inside themselves that their parent disliked them. Some very sensitive children—if they are constantly criticized—may develop a poor picture of themselves and never become vitalized or fully realized as adults because they are always doubting themselves. I do not see many of these children, but I do meet them when they have grown up, and they have had such histories. These are the people who are so drained of energy. I think we should keep our eyes out for such people and help them as we can.

Many sensitive children become self-centered because they develop a distrust of people. They feel or sense what a person means but it is not what that person is saying, and they do not know how to deal with it. If you can reach such a disturbed child and his parents, and for one minute project a sense of love, it would be helpful. Very often these children feel very alone, and just a bit of acceptance means a lot to them.

Don't hide the fact that the child might have picked up something. Always tell a child the truth; that is an important thing to consider with a sensitive child. If you accept that he has picked up someone's thoughts, you do him less damage than by putting him off and saying it never happened. You can simply say that he has picked up someone else's thoughts and it has nothing to do with him; let him know that such things do happen, then urge him to forget it. That is a sensible thing to say. I would make it commonplace.

You can say to the child, "It's all right. I know you are sorry. Let us just feel loving toward that person." These are simple words, but you are dealing with a sensitive child, and a child can do things an adult cannot. If a child touches your hands, for instance, and he or she looks up into your eyes, it makes an opening in your emotions in a very few minutes. You can let the child know in a very simple way that they can give joy to others, such as their parents, in this way; even that little bit of directing can be very helpful. Instead of feeling alone and lost, locked up in their feelings and unable to express them to others, they can release their emotions simply and directly through the heart-felt thought.

The same thing can happen, of course, with adults who touch those in need. Sometimes the momentary touching means a lot. It tells people who feel lost and fearful that they are not alone in the world, and it can be the most helpful thing to do under the circumstances.

I am trying to remember what happened in my case, for it was a very long time ago. I do remember that when I was a child I picked up if there was violence between people. I understood what it was, and so I went to the next room. I knew what people were feeling, and I did not like it, for it made me uncomfortable, but, as a little girl, I could do nothing about it. Therefore I decided that going away from that disruptive situation was the sensible thing to do.

In the case of deeply disturbed children, I first of all suggest that you do not have grandiose ideas. If you are doing TT to such a child, stand behind him and just make him feel peaceful. With TT you can reduce his stress in a few minutes, and you can then quietly talk to him.

That may be all you can do. Some children will respond, and some are so caught up in the violence that they are themselves out of control and cannot respond. You cannot help everybody. They do not necessarily want to be helped; but if you unobtrusively project a calm energy, invariably they will calm down in a few minutes. Then you can approach and help them.

One year we had a very disturbed little girl about two years old at one of our Therapeutic Touch workshops. I treated her, and she took a great fancy to me. She took my hand, and we went for a walk. Even though you cannot talk to a little child of two, nevertheless she quieted down, and never had the temper tantrum her parents expected. She was an oversensitive child and somewhat retarded. When I healed her, her sensitivity was not violated. I relaxed her, and she calmed down and responded to the healing. For one moment she felt calm and peaceful, and accepted. In that moment our inner selves met, and I could project a sense of calmness from that level. For the three or four days she stayed with us, she was a different child, with not a sign of her previous tantrums. Something had happened because of her great sensitivity, which picked up that everyone accepted her, and it had a lasting effect.

As sensitive children grow into adulthood, some of their sensitivity may persist, but the important thing is that over time they learn how to deal with it. I have spoken to many sensitive adults who, on the whole, are bothered by the sensitivity quite often, but they can rationalize it and therefore deal with the circumstances better than they could as children. For instance, if they are dealing with a personal problem and they pick up antagonism in somebody else, it does hurt. At such times I would suggest that they say to themselves, "All right, I accept it, and let me turn the situation around positively by sending that person a thought of goodwill." That positive response will break the negative projection. Some sensitive people are hypersensitive, and they are often wrong about the degree of what they pick up. They are sometimes led to exaggerate what they are perceiving because they don't have a sense of security within themselves.

Development of Self-Image

I do not think we understand the power of our consciousness and how it can hold us for many years in certain patterns that may damage us. The subtle energetic patterns we build by the way we repeatedly use our consciousness can control our lives without our being aware of it. By patterns I mean how we can get an idea, stick with that idea, and yet be unconscious that we are stuck with this one idea that we developed perhaps many years before. It can make us unhappy for the rest of our life, and we do not know what it is that makes us unhappy. It is a major problem for us today. We could call some part of this "memory," but I would like to tell you, from my point of view, how it works.

Whenever you have thoughts about yourself, they build up a picture—your interpretation of yourself—in the atmosphere around you. The picture you reflect on has a powerful effect. Responding repeatedly to this self-made picture creates a habit pattern that can affect your future life and what you think of yourself.

People often feel frustrated because, for instance, they cannot do things well, they cannot follow through on what they wish to do, and so forth. Not infrequently this gives rise to a feeling about themselves that they are not of much good. Such lack of self-confidence hurts a lot of children. We often fail to realize how this might affect a child in a negative way early in life. It has a powerful influence and can result in their carrying a negative picture of the self within them throughout their life. If they are at the same time driven by a picture of themselves as being very successful and try to do everything to bring about that success, they may significantly deplete their energy in the process.

We do not realize that our minds are conditioned early in life. We then get set along certain lines of thinking that make us absolutely certain about particular ideas; we see only one truth and everything else is wrong. Children in many parts of the country are brought up that way. That is sad because it is by listening that we keep our minds open. You do not have to argue with what people say, but by keeping your mind open you can learn about new facets of something in which you are interested. Many close their mind to an exchange of ideas. When this rigidity persists, it may lead to mental illness.

The Power of Energy Exchanges

Learning about the various levels of consciousness and how they react in our lives enables us to deal with problems revolving around consciousness in daily life. Frequently our feelings and thinking work together; more often in our culture they interfere with one another, such as when we feel something very strongly, and thoughtful consideration tells us that releasing the strong emotion is not a good idea. When thought interrupts our behavior, it may bring us into conflict in ourselves; we may have many battles of indecision going on within us. Further, these conflicts can then affect our physical body, often without our realizing that there is this connection.

We need to realize that within us we have these different aspects, and that sometimes our emotions and our life experiences make us very confused and unhappy. As a result, we block the energy of the inner self, and it is no longer active within us. If we get caught in the blind strength of our feelings at the emotional level, it not only affects the part of our mind that is working closely with our emotions; it can even block certain aspects of the level of pure thinking. The intuitional level, however, is not usually completely blocked. It is always there, and sometimes we get a clear insight that profoundly affects our emotions and our thinking, often offering ideas on how to resolve the conflict or other emotional upset.

All these interior interactions, you must remember, are part of your inner self. This is often difficult for most people to accept. Although the inner self has energetic characteristics of peace and quiet, when we give ourselves over to inner dynamics of thoughts and feelings in conflict, the conflict blocks the influence of the inner self that is normally streaming through the various levels of consciousness. It is this influence that lends considerable strength to our ability to carry out our ideas in the physical world, but the turmoil of the conflict stifles it.

In a very real way your negative thoughts or emotions feed back powerfully on yourself. How that happens is this: you send out a negative thought and your subconscious mind realizes that it is negative or unhelpful to the recipient of that thought, so you are ambivalent, usually not realizing at all what is happening. It may not make sense to you, but from my point of view, the energy involved in the incident strengthens your ambivalence and makes you feel worse. This emotional disturbance then hooks into the reverse effect or feedback.

If you happen to be doing Therapeutic Touch at that time, there is the possibility that during the assessment you may attribute your emotional disturbance to the patient or you might project that negative load onto them during the rebalancing. When you first begin to center preparatory to doing Therapeutic Touch, if you could take a moment and realize that you are trying to be in harmony with all living things, not only the patient, and include the patient within that sense of harmony, that would give you a different perspective, and it would also help to release your pent-up emotions in a constructive way. If you take the time to center, you probably will pick up the problem and might be of help to that person.

We do not realize the power of our feelings as an energy field that affects others, more so in our everyday affairs than when we are doing Therapeutic Touch. We are sending messages to our children, other members of our family, other persons in our immediate circle of friends and colleagues, and in some cases, perfect strangers who may interact with us in our daily activities. Many people I see have difficult lives because they are not aware that energy exchanges are constantly taking place between themselves and others, significantly, although unconsciously, affecting them. It is important to realize that you can respond in a positive manner or, on the other hand, how such energy exchanges can act to disturb your mind.

Recently a young woman came to me. She had a very good job, but she hated her boss. In spite of an opportunity to be promoted, she could not stand him. She said, "He makes me so nervous that I think I have to give it up." I told her to go to work a few minutes early each day, arriving before her boss got in. She was just to calm herself, and when her boss came in she would simply send him a sense of goodwill. She started each day with intentionally sending him a quiet energy—before they clashed. In two month's time she told me that everything had changed. He no longer had the outbursts of temper. He had confided in her that he had intense physical pain and was very worried about it. In all the years she had worked next to him she had thought that he was a nasty man. She said that their relationship had worked out because she had learned to listen to him. Sending goodwill, which she continued to do, in some way rested him and he seemed much calmer. The relationship strengthened, and she continued in that job.

This is a simple story, but I want you to realize, without putting a value on emotions, that we are constantly exchanging energies with people in our relationships. We aren't just talking to one another; we are actually exchanging energy. Thus, even if we do not say one word, we can send energy that can help, for instance, to balance a relationship, or to calm an agitated person. On the other hand, if another person gets irritated with you constantly, it is important to recognize that there is the chance that you are being filled with the ceaseless streaming of irritation that is being directed toward you.

I have dealt with many people who are mentally ill. They feel and think in certain ways, but they feel it inside of themselves. When you and I have or come in touch with an emotion or thought that we do not feel is healthy or that we do not like, we have the capacity to reject it or talk it over with someone else and then let it go. This capacity of expanding upon it in thought or word and throwing it out is not functioning fully in those who are mentally ill. Because their feelings stay within them, much of their energy flow automatically encloses in on them instead of going outward. This is part of their sickness. Instead of being released, the energy comes back upon them and reinforces their inability to flow out into the world and have an exchange with others. The complete inward-turning of a person's energy flow makes them lonelier and increases their mental strain. If we can help them break through their self-made barrier of constantly feeding on their own emotions, they could feel interactions with others and make relationships again, and that would be constructive and helpful.

All of us have the need to have our feelings flow outward and interact with others; it is a law of Nature. We do not often think of the basic need people have for that kind of exchange, that ability to go out to someone or something. The need for this kind of outlet is great in our society at this time. So many people are turning inward, even young people, and all of us can help. Recommendations or suggestions of the simplest kind often work.

In large cities, many people are very lonely. I remember meeting a very poor woman who lived in a housing project in New York City. What came to mind was to suggest to her that she get a cat. She followed my advice and got a cat and came back to see me three months later. She had a smile on her face; she was a different person, a happier person, because she was living with something with which she could interact. A cat seems a simple thing, but the opportunity to interact with a living being made a tremendous difference to this lady. That something returned her affection and that she could give that affection meant so much in her life.

A cat may be the answer for one person, a plant that the person has to nourish may work for another. You want to help them find an opportunity to get outside of themselves and perhaps form a relationship and have interactions with the outer world, even in the simplest way. So many people have no outlet and if you can provide that in any way, you can be of significant help.

The Effect of Mind-Pictures

Our feelings and our thinking combined have a strong influence upon us. One of their aspects, memory, has a profound effect on our behavior. If you repeat something over and over again in your memory that happened when you were a child or a youth, you may connect that event with a picture of a person who was associated with the original event. For many years you may do very well, but within yourself, at the emotional level of consciousness, you build up resentment toward that image. You send the resentment to the person in that picture, and those energies serve to feed, or strengthen, the picture you have built in your emotional field. Also, when you feel even slightly resentful about other things that may not be of great importance in themselves, their emotional energies also go directly to that picture you have formed. Resentment is a kind of hatred, one of the most powerful bonds, and you are linking yourself to that through your memories.

Most of us are willing to accept that our emotions affect us, but not so many will accept that our mind-pictures affect us. Mind-pictures, of course, are memories, and memories are a force acting on us energetically, even physiologically. When you think of a mind-picture of something that occurred in the past, perhaps something fearful, you once again have a similar feeling of fear or lack of self-confidence. The associations with that picture have several facets, but many times you are not aware of this; you do not make the connection to that time long ago. Nevertheless, the mind-pictures have gained strength as you repeatedly remembered them, and this repetitious recall serves to reinforce the lack of confidence or the fear.

The only reality of that memory is that you, yourself, are hanging onto it and giving it life; you may not be recognizing that you have grown beyond that thought. In other words, the person who is still holding resentment has changed through the years, and the object of that resentment is also a very different person, perhaps having grown in insight, and so the resentful thought no longer has a reality base. Holding on to a thought of a relationship brings out in oneself a lot of resentment and anger and the memory affects one's perspective of life. This phenomenon is very much like the mind-picture a sick person harbors about his illness.

If you do this, in one sense the inner self has to accept it, for it cannot interfere with your free choice. The personality is born with certain capacities and has to develop by itself. You would not learn and grow if the inner self constantly interfered. So the inner self also has to accept that you are binding yourself to a memory of resentment. Nevertheless, under dire circumstances the individual can get help from the inner self, if it is appropriate.

I have met people who have held bitter resentment for twenty or thirty years because they feel they have been thwarted. What they do not realize is that they are holding themselves back. They are not aware of their own life changes during that time. I think spending twenty or thirty years dissecting memories of one's earlier life is a lot of time to invest in events that have passed.

What I want to impress upon you is the realization that when any of us carry such fear or resentments, we are building our present attitudes or behaviors on a past that has nothing to do with us as mature adults. It is not so hard to change, if we realize that some of our feelings lie within our memory and may no longer be part of our present way of life. We can say: "All right, this is a memory of something in my past. I am through with it. I am not bound by it any longer. I am living today, at this moment, *in the present.*" Then, when we automatically want to return to that picture of helplessness, we will instead see ourselves as strong and realize that it is not necessary to get caught up in that memory again. I do not say that this is easy to do, but it can be done, and it can have a life-changing effect.

The Use and Abuse of Memory

This understanding of the power of mind-pictures can be used to help people who have been abused as children. Certain people are brought up with the idea that it is perfectly right to hit and punish their children. The idea that this kind of behavior is all right pervades the cultures of certain groups and has been accepted for hundreds of years, but today we live in a different world. Still, that idea has been exaggerated, particularly among those who need a sense of control, and among those who do not reflect upon the consequences, resulting in an incredible amount of child abuse today.

The problem of abuse in today's culture comes up time and again in the work that I do. It is the focusing on it—the effect of the persevering memory—that is at the core of the problem. One thing that people forget about abused children is that when they were abused they were, in fact, children, and that they were helpless. They were not strong and they had to endure it. When they become adults they retain the memory of those long-past events and associate the child who was helpless with their present self. It seems a pity that so many people with such extremely painful memories still hang on to such depressing thoughts. By perpetuating that picture of themselves, they hold on to their resentment and they are also prevented from having a normal level of self-confidence.

I do not think that the medical profession realizes that the sense of helplessness of those who are abused—being fired over time by resentment—reverberates over their lifetime, never allowing them to feel self-confident. They need a positive therapy that helps the abused person to realize that it happened a long time ago and to recognize that they are now strong and grown up and reacting to a memory only. Frequently they have built a wall around the memory itself and the strength of their emotions adds to the pent-up energies connected with it. Through the interaction of the recall of the abuse and the associated feelings, what they remember is often exaggerated. In many avenues of psychotherapy, patients are encouraged to remember all this and bring it back to the therapy session. The pity of this is that they are not coming to grips with the problem itself.

The basic problem is not only the lack of self-confidence or the fear, but the original inability to deal with the abuse. I would think that the pain and the actual events have probably faded and what they are left with is a sense of helplessness: there was an effect on their life that they could not control. Often it is a parent who has caused the abuse, and frequently the abused persons will say that they have forgiven those who have abused them. But they are fooling themselves; forgiveness has not really been given. These are just words, and they are meaningless. The tie to what happened has not been broken; the memory of the incidents and their various associations keep returning, because forgiveness has not truly taken place. This continued association with the experience is at the heart of the person's present problem and it must be recognized.

When I counsel people who have been abused as children, the first thing I point out is that they are now strong and independent, but are living with the *memory* of helplessness. I think we may often fail to bring that point to the attention of the one who has been abused or the person harboring resentment. When they grow up, they are no longer helpless: that is the crucial acknowledgement. I suggest that they recognize and actually say to themselves, "I am my own person; I am grown up; I am *not* helpless now," and that they forget that at one time they were. That last phrase may sound contrived to you, but the fact is that they are not helpless and the incident is in the past. I think that before they can get rid of that problem, they must acknowledge what they are today.

I also teach people who have been abused or who hold resentment the importance of breaking their image of resentment. They have built up a picture of the person or event that has hurt them so much. In reality, part of them is attached to that. They do not accept that something upsetting has happened in the past, nor do they recognize that they are keeping alive that relationship or the image of suffering, which is now actually a reaction on their part and not a true relationship between two or more people. From my point of view, the impression of suffering is kept alive because they are hanging on to that image.

Instead, they could say—and this is a hard thing to say—"Am I the same person?" If they are honest with themselves, they will see that they are a different person from when the incident occurred, that time has passed, and that what they are hanging onto and giving energy to is but a memory of their suffering, a memory that they have built. If they can do this, the relationship will be changed, and even the memory will not be so painful.

Each of us is more easily upset by different situations, but we all are upset by suffering. I would not put a time limit on how long suffering actually lasts. It may be weeks, months, or years; however, many people feel they have been suffering all their lives. Now, their memory of suffering may last a lifetime, but the acute period rarely lasts more than a few to several months. If we suffer, or are in the presence of other people who are suffering, we can rely on one thing: the suffering will last only for a short time, although to the sufferer it will seem like an eternity and he will not believe it will ever be over. In such a circumstance, if we could for one minute think of the quietness of the inner self, it would help us to see and to convey that nothing really lasts for very long.

When we get into a healing relationship and recognize that a patient holds resentment toward someone else, it might be helpful to first let him talk about that relationship. Then help him to realize that the other person is a human being lost in his own difficulties. Emphasize to the patient that by thinking in this resentful way all the time, he is being hooked and that he is hurting himself; in fact, by holding the negative emotion, he is doing much more harm to himself than to the other person. If someone has a relationship that ends in resentment and anger, I think that is a very unfinished relationship. If one person in the relationship dies, it makes it very painful for those who are living to think of the person on the other side with such bitterness.

To help a person release his resentment, be very calm, nonjudgmental, and give him emotional support. If you are in a healing relationship, you cannot be judgmental because you are trying to perceive in the patient a touch of the inner self, and the real work of each person's inner self is truly beyond our understanding. For the person who holds resentment, it is almost as though he has built it into his thoughts, and these thoughts stay around him—hovering, brooding thoughts of resentment. The resentful person no longer thinks of the individual against whom he holds the resentment, he is so totally enclosed in his resentment. When a person is so imprisoned, he cannot have any fresh feelings. It is a very unhealthy climate to surround oneself with, and the quicker the person gets rid of it, the better; so we should help that person to do it.

Very importantly, he needs to become aware that he is binding himself. To free himself, he needs to first acknowledge his attachment to a bitter, negative habit pattern. You can tell your patient that the two binding forces are love and resentment, perhaps a few times, for he may not be listening to you the first time. If he really hears you, it will make an impression after a while. This can be effectively done during the Therapeutic Touch session as you reach out to the consciousness of the patient. Suggest that he reevaluate the situation, think of the person in the greater sense of their being a "whole person"—in reference to their own background and difficulties—and then send that person good will. Good will, not love, for you cannot tell someone who is full of resentment that he has to love somebody. In this instance, *love* would be a word to be very carefully avoided.

Patients are primarily concerned about themselves. They think about their pain; they fill their minds with memories of painful periods in the past; they constantly have in mind the prognosis and are under great strain. So, the most important thing is to begin by relaxing them. Ask them if they feel better and if they do, tell them, "These memories happened some time ago. You are alive *now*. Don't you think it is possible to change?" People do not realize how much they live in their memories and are not living now, in the present moment. It is a most important fact to bring to people's attention whether they are sick or well. It is surprising to find how many bad memories people have.

Therefore, confront them by asking, "Do you *want* to change?" If they do, they will give themselves wholeheartedly to change.

People who are convinced of their inner self know that they have the power to change; those who do not have this conviction can be taught that they can change by using the power of their mind or their will, however they conceive it. Then they can learn to reject this image with its accompanying load of resentful feelings. People *can* change; they are *not* powerless and they should be encouraged to use that capacity in their own lives. All schools of meditation suggest that you find some sense of peace within yourself. That is a universal quest. Concentrating on the idea that you can find peace within yourself is a positive approach. However, the idea of the inner self also means that you think of yourself as strong and that, to a certain extent, the power of change is within yourself. I do not think all schools of meditation stress that.

There are people who are completely carried away by their raging emotions again and again and these emotional storms can drain their energy. Many will not give up these bouts of fury because they are "hooked" (which is very descriptive of what these highly charged thoughts look like in their emotional field). Healing indicates change. If a person wants to be helped they must recognize this and want to change these violent reactions. Persons who are very sick often are willing to change, whereas those who are not so ill will resist changing their behavior. Those not willing to change will be harder to heal; nevertheless it is your duty to try. If they will not change, just help them to the best of your ability. Whether you succeed completely or not is not in your hands. It has to be the ill person's choice; it is not easy to give up a habit and the individual concerned must make the decision.

However, Therapeutic Touch is so different and so gentle, it may induce a person to be willing to change. Sometimes a harsh approach stimulates resistance, whereas gentleness eases a person into change. If you are doing TT right, you are calling upon a source that is not yourself, so you are not personally attached to the outcome of the therapeutic interaction. Also, when you do Therapeutic Touch to a person, over time you open them up a little bit to their inner self, from which they get intuitions and insights. If they are responsive, they begin to listen to their inner self. This has been very evident to me particularly among AIDS patients who have gone on to die. However, they have died peacefully, and those who work with such persons say that this is not so common.

Resolving Resentment in the Healer

Understanding this will help you, too, as TT therapist, wipe out your own prejudices as you try to reach out to others in compassion. After some time of practicing Therapeutic Touch, you get a grasp on your intuitions and you act, automatically doing the right thing. You may not even think about it; you get the perception of what is the right thing to do, and you do it. That comes with considerable practice and experience. But you may still be caught by your mind-pictures and an associated sense of helplessness.

To treat this problem therapeutically, you must first become aware of the prejudice or the resentment. Most often we are completely unaware of our prejudgments, even in families. There may be a feeling of unease, particularly if you are a sensitive person. In general, however, most people are unaware of this on-going process and, even if they feel the reaction, quickly forget it. Once you have understood the strength of your emotions and your thoughts, you can recognize that if you feel resentment to a parent or other person, you remain tied them if you have never worked out that relationship. You can deal with this by first of all acknowledging that you have hooked into a painful memory from your past, and then firmly asserting, "I want to be rid of it; I am living *now!*" That is a very strong concept you must build. You have to break through those ambivalences. You do not want to continue coming back to that mind-picture with its overtones of helplessness.

Resentment is human; however, in healing, resentment stops you from becoming a complete healer. As a healer, you must be open, and so the energy cannot be blocked as it will be if resentment is allowed to fester. Strong emotional patterns such as resentment take time to build, and they are difficult to change. But the idea that you have an inner self, that you have an integrating power, can help you to forge ahead in life. I suggest that resentful people do the following exercise for at least two or three months; that much time is needed to do this successfully.

୧ᓎᓎ Suggested Exercise to ᓎᓎ
Resolve Resentment

If you can learn to be quiet within yourself and then think of the person you have resentment toward, think of him as being some distance away. Visualize that person for two or three minutes, but do not associate the name or symbol of father, mother, or any kind of relationship with the visualization. Think of him neutrally, as a human being, with a personal inner self in his own right. If you can think of him as that inner self, send him a feeling of goodwill. I am not saying "love," remember that; however, you could send goodwill.

If you really say "I will do it," the personal commitment, "I," will draw on the power of your inner self. When you experience this process, if you then go into TT or meditation, you will feel much freer; something will have been released from the background of your mind. You will have strengthened your relationship with your inner self. In this way you are achieving something, not just at the emotional level, but on all the levels of consciousness. It is not easy, but it will give you peace of mind, and it is one way of breaking these unconscious patterns. You are breaking with the past and can now form a new relationship. Perhaps you will not believe this, but it does reach the person, and it may help him to re-evaluate his behavior.

I want to emphasize that I am not speaking here of sending forgiveness or love, but goodwill. There is a difference between them. It is unrealistic to expect yourself (or anyone) to love a person you resent; however, sending good will is possible. Even if you have a tremendous resentment, it would not be so hard to send a neutral thought such as goodwill every morning, because even if you do not like the person, you do want him to go on with his own spiritual evolution. You do not know but that person is suffering in his own way. Do it as a form of discipline for two months. It is a different way of thinking.

People to whom I have taught this have phoned me to say that after several months their strongly focused thoughts had reached the person they had previously resented. They knew this because that person had contacted them. They told me that even though there had been no communication for the previous two or three years, the relationship was now changed. They freed themselves from their bondage to the resentment.

If you can do this, you can lose forever the sense of helplessness that is associated with that memory. You come in at another level, as the giver. The moment you can do that, the memory will change. It is not easy to do, but it can be done. It might be good to avoid having any communications with the person for whom you hold resentment for the two or three months you are doing this exercise. You have to work out this inner relationship on your own. You will need the two months; it must be done in complete freedom from time constraints and other pressures. Interaction with that person will make you feel ambivalent. You see the phone, and even if you are thousands of miles from the person, it can act as an irritant, a constant reminder. If you allow that reflex to recur, it will stop the healing process. In the first two months you must be resolute; when you feel free of it, it will not bother you.

Parents very often have a lot of things to work out too, and frequently they will pick on the nearest child to share the moments when they are irritated. When it is a case of abuse, it is like salt in a wound to the child. As a child of such parents, if you can be free from this for two or more months during the exercise, it will help you to maintain your balance. After a few months, if you have to be on the phone with the person with whom you are having the problem, simply say, "I am sorry; I do think of you," if you have to explain why you have not been in touch, but do not have very long phone calls, unless there can be a friendly exchange and you have something meaningful to say to each other.

☙ Breaking Out of Negative ❧
Emotional Cycles

What you do not want to do is to pick up the anxiety of the person on the other end of the phone connection, or to deepen your resentment, if he or she is trying to hurt your feelings.

Center yourself and send him blue, a sense of peace. The moment you can do that you are protecting yourself against the intake of the negativity that has been projected by that person. Instead of opening yourself up to his negative thoughts and becoming more and more resentful as the conversation goes on, talk for a short time, say whatever you have to say, and get off the phone. One can break the negative cycle without becoming irritated or further resentful, by remembering to bring the consciousness to center, so that you can once again be in touch with your inner self. That will help you in your resolve.

If someone is feeling resentful to you, you can do something similar to help resolve the situation. Sometimes there is nothing you can do. However the possibility is worth the try. Do not listen to what the person carrying the resentment says, because most frequently the reaction is to exaggerate what they have suffered. Instead, turn inward and feel the peace and strength within yourself. That indication of personal integrity probably would surprise the other person too. Then quietly but deliberately send him a sense of goodwill and see if it penetrates. Remember that you must, first of all, have a period when you withdraw within yourself, and then you send the goodwill. You are not expecting anything from the other person; you just want to have a peaceful relationship. It is a kind of nonattachment, of course.

If the other person's resentment turns verbally abusive, you must find the courage to quietly say aloud, "I'm not going to stand for that abuse anymore. Do you realize that?" In this way the message comes across intellectually as well as emotionally. To do this you must have self-confidence, a sense of the reality of your inner self. A useful mantra to say to oneself is, "I am that self." Then you can make the statement that you are not going to stand for that abuse anymore. If you cannot confront the person, write him a letter, explaining in detail what you are going to do. If the person understands what you are saying, it will change the way he sees you and may change the relationship. Then you can make the final decision on the right course to proceed.

CHAKRAS AND THE THERAPEUTIC TOUCH PROCESS

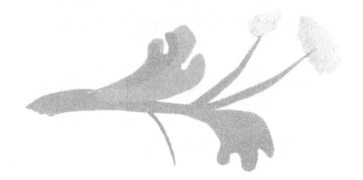

Introductory Comments

The idea that nonphysical complexes of patterned subtle energies form centers for the different kinds of human consciousness is deeply embedded in the histories of diverse cultures. Such indications occur in Central America, in an ancient text, the Popul Vuh; in the Near East, among the Sufis; in the southwestern United States, among the Apaches, the Hopi, and the Zuni peoples; and among the Huna of Hawaii. It also forms an important part of the belief systems of the people of Asia, most notably among the Tibetans, the Japanese, the Chinese, and in India, where this knowledge is discussed in detail in the Upanishads, which are part of the most ancient literature of the Hindus, the Vedas.

In the development of Therapeutic Touch, we have chosen to relate to the Indian version, whose approach appeals most to the modern Western mind. In Indian philosophy, these centers of consciousness are called chakras, a Sanskrit term that has come into the popular English idiom in the past quarter century. Dora Kunz was considered a foremost authority on the subtle energy dynamics of the chakras, and it was her expertise that allowed us to develop Therapeutic Touch as a safe and profound practice. In Therapeutic Touch we usually work with the upper chakras; that is, those that have a physiological reference from the solar plexus upward toward the head of the body.

However, by far the major chakra the TT therapist relates to is the heart chakra, for a number of reasons. It has been mentioned that entry into the Therapeutic Touch process is through the centering of one's consciousness in the heart. Because the heart chakra is the locus where the act of centering is sustained, all aspects of the Therapeutic Touch process go through it. The heart chakra is functionally affiliated with both the vital-energy field, where it is concerned with such critical functions as the circulation of the of the blood and the maintenance of blood pressure, and the psychodynamic field, which is involved with psychological behaviors, many of them expressing altruistic and humane attributes, such as love and compassion. The compassion that initiates the act of helping or healing someone in need is one of the major properties of the heart chakra. Interestingly, the Upanishad states that there is a close connection between the heart chakra and the hand chakras, which form a central part of the techniques of Therapeutic Touch.

Within the chakra complex, the heart chakra is very closely connected to both the brow chakra and the crown chakra and, as Dora notes in this section, the heart chakra is the most physical site from which the inner self enters into the daily activities of living.

These items of information detail an important part of the logic that Dora and I followed in the development of Therapeutic Touch, and indicate why TT can operate with considerable safety and at a significant depth for the healee while exerting a singular life-affirmative effect on both healer and healee. They clarify how this gentle art of compassion can actually force positive transformation in those who practice it.

The Chakras as Centers
of Consciousness

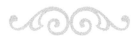

THE CONCEPT OF CHAKRAS AS CENTERS OF CONSCIOUSNESS has been accepted for thousands of years, particularly in the Hindu tradition. While I personally was brought up on the idea of chakras, discussion about them has recently become very popular. In this section I shall describe some of the characteristics of chakras and their relationship to the Therapeutic Touch process.

The chakras are centers of subtle energies that are closely related to the physical body and, therefore, are associated with human disease processes. The brain and the chakras act throughout a person's lifetime. They die with the physical body, and I think eventually the chakras themselves disappear. But it is important to remember that these centers are basically part of consciousness, the one thing that acts unceasingly. Consciousness dominates everything we do, so there is always a coordinated connection between the chakras. They show our different spiritual capacities and our mental capacities, if they are developed.

Chakras have been described as wheels that are constantly revolving in the subtle energy fields of a person. One of their important characteristics is that they each have their own intrinsic rhythm, but there is an integrated rhythm all over the body. Often it is this rhythm that goes out of balance when a person is ill. Certain colors and tones are associated with each of the chakras, although the tones are less readily perceivable than the colorations. Under certain circumstances, the colors sometimes change as they turn around; it is almost as if the light goes through them.

Nothing in the world is separate and there is nothing that does not interact. There are slightly different levels of energy, but they all interact together. We often do not realize that at the same time the flows of our various senses bring us information, they also affect the energy of our physical body. For instance, if you are outside among the trees, getting pleasure out of looking at them, that experience fills you with energy. It is a positive interaction between you and the beautiful trees and it adds to your sense of well being. The chakras in the subtle energy fields act as transformers for these different levels of energy. The energies interpenetrate each other, and the chakras move within the body in a rhythmic and integrated way. They form a unified and dynamic whole in which, for example, our thoughts affect our emotions, and our emotions affect our physical body. The human constitution functions at all these levels of consciousness.

The crown chakra, located on the top of the head, is the largest and one of the most central of the chakras. It is involved in an integrated energetic relationship with all of the rest of the chakras. The crown chakra has a core surrounded by what you could call flower petals or the spokes of a wheel, which also turn around. It is not really a wheel, because a wheel is closed and the chakra is not closed. It deals with consciousness and is very closely associated with the brain. This chakra affects everything we do, because the brain is central to all behavior, determining how we see the world and how we interpret it. The pineal is an important gland that has a very close relationship with the crown chakra.

There is a much smaller center ascribed to the middle of the forehead, often called the brow chakra or the third eye. This center has several functions, as it is associated with thinking, perception, and clairvoyance. I think it is also connected with the brain and the pituitary. It is concerned with how the individual sees things, but also with the flashes of intuition and the brain's interpretation of them. There is a very close relationship between the crown and the brow chakras at subtle energy levels. After all, our visual perception physically is very closely linked to the brain. A person who thinks very clearly may get flashes of intuition, perhaps with a visual image, when the two chakras get together in harmony. When the brow chakra is active, it is more illuminated and its rhythm is different from the other centers. If a person is clairvoyant, its rhythm—the way it moves through space—is faster.

The next center of consciousness is the same size, more or less, as the brow chakra. It is at the throat, the instrument for the voice. Major functions of this chakra concern energy, rhythm, and sound. The throat chakra has a great deal to do with a person's sensitivity to sound, not necessarily sound the way we understand it, but harmonic sound. We see this sensitivity not only in people who are interested in music, but also in those who are interested in rhythm. The throat chakra is greatly developed in dancers and musicians. Of course, this chakra also has an association with what we call the thyroid.

Next, one comes down to the heart chakra. Like consciousness, the heart is vital for our existence. The heart chakra processes our aspirations, our genuine affection, love, and compassion with nonattachment to the outcome. The heart chakra is really the center of our existence. It is closest to being the center of consciousness of the inner self in the physical body, so psychic sensitivity also has its center here. This center is well developed in people who do a great deal of meditation. In addition, it is also a major center of balance. Three chakras—the heart, the brow, and the crown—work closely together. Although this is difficult to comprehend, there is a perfectly healthy steady relationship in the rhythm and exchange of energy between all these chakras as they turn around.

The heart is a link between the emotional and the physical levels of consciousness. To a certain extent the rhythm of the heart and the emotions are related. For example, when you feel upset—in the grip of a strong feeling or by picking up other people's feelings—the emotional energy of your body is brought into your awareness (in the brain) through your heart, which solely has to do with your physical body. The thymus—located near the center of the chest and related to the immune system—is also within the sphere of influence of the heart chakra.

The next chakra to be considered is related to the solar plexus. One of the largest chakras, it has to do with one's feelings and it is the center of the body's energy systems: the adrenals, the stomach, and digestive functions. Likes, dislikes, anger—all these emotions go through the solar plexus chakra, and dysfunction of the associated organs can result when they are negatively charged. Because the emotions are so definitely involved, this chakra and the heart chakra work very closely together.

The rhythm of the solar plexus chakra changes more often than that of the others; it is probably the chakra that is the most affected by daily living. When people are sick, there is always a lot of disturbance in their solar plexus chakra. Many people get sick physically and emotionally; most have an emotional disturbance about being sick. Even in a person with a mild sickness and without much emotional disturbance, this chakra is a little out of kilter. If a person gets very emotionally upset, something that lasts several days, it can get out of rhythm and the person may get an upset stomach. If the physical dysfunctions that stem from such a continued state develop, it is here that one finds clues to the problem, which may take the form of emotional imbalance, or of psychosomatic illnesses. The condition, if prolonged, can go on to do organic damage, such as occurs with peptic ulcers. I have met some of the patients in mental institutions, and can confirm that there is a relation between disturbed feelings and the dysrhythmia of this chakra.

When a person is in a healthy state, the solar plexus chakra is functioning in a balanced manner. If such a person could go into a room of persons who are very ill and remain quiet and centered, that individual would be the ideal person to do Therapeutic Touch. Such a person is capable of calmly and helpfully relating to pain and anguish in others without first relating to an agenda of personal needs.

There is also a minor chakra related to the spleen. It absorbs energy from sunlight, as *prana,* and functions to energize the whole body. Science is now finding this interaction to be of vital importance to physical health. Chronic fatigue syndrome is one indication of a malfunction of this chakra. It also goes out of kilter in a person with a serious illness, causing a lowered absorption of life-energy.

At the base of the spine is a large chakra, the root chakra, about which most of us know very little. It is very powerful. This is where one finds the energy called *kundalini,* which in its developed form has to do with spiritual attainment, and is closely connected to the brain. Its major functions do not have so much to do with physical health as with binding all the chakras together so that they function as one. If one does a great deal of meditation and adheres to a spiritual discipline, this energy—which is usually dormant—may rise and become active. This may happen if a person is really committed to a particular style of living or philosophy and acts it out.

Even though *kundalini* energy is not very active in most people, the spinal cord itself is still very active and is connected with many of our physical organs and functions. The energies coming from the chakras flow through the entire spine, so that consciousness itself radiates everywhere. The spine is not individually connected to a chakra; the chakras are all linked together, and so they dynamically relate to one another.

There are very small centers in the hands; we can't really call them chakras, but we can call them centers of consciousness. It is because of them that you can project healing through your hands when you do TT. Your hands are connectors to send energy visualized by your mind. You are using yourself as a transmitter, but your mind is also concerned with the intentionality of your healing.

There are also chakras in the feet. When we walk on the Earth, these centers are in touch with the tremendous amount of energy in the Earth. If we meditate, and if we are doing TT properly, we tap into that energy. I think the feet also help to eliminate negative feelings. A person who is full of negative emotional pain can think of the energy going out through their feet and into the Earth. It will not hurt the Earth.

Clinical Relationships
to the Chakras

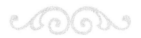

Overview

NOW, WHAT IS THE PURPOSE of what I have described? How do the chakras relate to disease? These centers of energy and consciousness are part of the natural process of our vital-energy field. They are individual but related systems that have to do with our bodily functions. When the body is ill, they individually or collectively get out of rhythm, and that dysrhythmia affects the whole body. In the Therapeutic Touch process, some of the higher, more subtle energies enter these centers and affect the physical body. Healing is a natural process, so it will work whether or not the persons involved are aware of the functioning of the chakras.

Many years ago, I made friends with Dr. Shafica Karagulla. When I first met her, she was very skeptical about such things, but she asked me to work with her. She wanted me to use my abilities to look at the chakras of her patients and describe them so that she could see if there was a relationship between my descriptions and their medical diagnoses. Based on this work, we wrote *The Chakras and the Human Energy Fields* (Karagulla and Kunz, 1989), in which I described the chakras of all the patients I saw with Dr. Karagulla and she discussed how my observations related to her diagnoses.

Dr. Karagulla had worked with Dr. Wilder Penfield, a very famous neurosurgeon in Canada, who had performed the first brain surgery operations on epileptics. As the result of her many years of work with Dr. Penfield, Dr. Karagulla became very interested in epilepsy and brain surgery. She asked me to observe some of Dr. Penfield's patients who were in New York City. When I first started working with Dr. Karagulla, I did not know that the people I was observing were epileptics; I did not know any of their conditions or even their names.

In my work with Dr. Karagulla, I described the disrupted functioning of the chakras I observed. As they turned around, I described where they appeared to be in perfect shape and where they appeared to be damaged. Frequently, part of the chakra was working, but the rhythm was not synchronized. Most of the people I wrote about in *The Chakras and the Human Energy Fields* had had epilepsy and other neural diseases for many years, so I was describing chronic states.

Without a doubt, certain diseases distort the motion of the chakras, such as causing them to rotate in opposite directions from their normal rotation. Some of the chakras of people who are mentally ill may also be out of kilter, the rhythm not functioning properly in certain parts of those energy centers. There are also people who are born with malfunctioning energy centers, for instance in inherited disease. Severe chronic diseases that have gone on for a long time may have a similar effect of upsetting the rhythm of some of the chakras, so that the abnormal intake of energy keeps the disease functioning longer.

I want to correct a misconception—conveyed by many books—that disease starts in the chakras. Diseases are physical. A person gets a disease, and *then* the chakras are affected. There may be emotional disturbances that contribute to the continuing disorder of the chakras, but the disease does not originate in the chakras. When the physical condition changes, the chakras go back to the way they should be; their disruption is not permanent. If you have a headache for one day, that is not going to affect your chakras. But if you have a genuine disease process, the vitality of your whole body is impacted, and that also affects the different chakras.

The chakras, of course, are connected with our physical organs. When a physical organ that is related to a particular chakra is operated upon, the energy of the chakra is depleted and this is seen as profound fatigue in the person post-surgically. Such patients can be helped by Therapeutic Touch if it is done very gently and rhythmically, while the therapist quietly maintains her own inner balance. *Nature* magazine recently published the results of studies regarding the impact of TT on patients undergoing heart surgery. When TT was done before surgery with emphasis on the heart, the patient remained very quiet and relaxed during the surgery and post-surgery. Moreover, the study found, these patients were released from the hospital two days earlier than was expected and they were in very good health.

People tell me that some healing modalities or books about chakras suggest that it is dangerous to open the chakras. I believe all of this discussion about opening and closing chakras is nonsense. You could not "open" a chakra if you wanted to. Chakras are mostly always open; after all, they have to have access to energy to function. I have never known a chakra to be shut. If there is a severe disease, I think you could say they are actually more open. If patients are very sick, it is more accurate to say that the chakras do not function very well. It is possible to add more energy to a chakra, but you don't have to be concerned about putting too much energy because the chakras know how to behave and regulate themselves. Meditative practices do, I believe, have an effect on one's chakras, particularly in altering their rhythms to some degree, but rhythmicity is only one aspect of their complexity. I do not think that the average person can alter the chakras of other persons, and it is just as well, for they have a multitude of effects on the body.

Crown Chakra

I did most of my work with Dr. Karagulla on the crown chakra because epilepsy and brain tumors are conditions that reflect dysfunctions of consciousness. I do not think that most of us realize—even though we may have read it in a textbook—how closely the brain and consciousness work together. They are inseparable. If there is something wrong with the brain, it is reflected in this chakra. If you get a disease like epilepsy—the major illness related to consciousness—the rhythm of the chakra gets disrupted. Here again I want to emphasize that *the chakra does not have the disease,* but is affected by the disease. I think that is a very different point of view and needs to be emphasized because it is vital to a true understanding of chakra function. If a person is perfectly healthy, the crown chakra will turn regularly.

The lowest level of consciousness energizes our physical system.

Our thinking is involved in that particular energy, which in the theosophical tradition is called the etheric. The crown chakra manifests first at the physical level, and that is why it is closely related to the brain function. The brain, as an organ, has its own system. It is a very complicated piece of machinery, the most complicated piece of machinery we have in our body. Its impact is very far reaching, affecting the whole of the body and an enormous number of its functions.

An epileptic seizure is caused by the brain function. In turn, the seizure causes a change in the person's level of consciousness for a second or a few minutes. I am able to see that it also affects the turning point and the rhythm of the crown chakra. If consciousness is constantly interrupted—such as in some of Dr. Penfield's patients who had seizures every five minutes—some of the petals or the spokes of the chakra also are affected. Dr. Penfield removed part of the brain of such patients and their symptoms of epilepsy disappeared, at least for a while. In many of the post-op patients I saw, the crown chakra behaved normally, but in others, it had a remnant of dysfunction.

When I have a patient before me, I know where the disease is because I perceive it directly, and I try to send healing energy that will bring order to the disordered part of the affected field. From my perspective—regarding the functioning of the chakra—epilepsy is an imbalance and not an actual disease. In treating the brain with Therapeutic Touch, one has to be very careful, because it cannot take too much energy. The brain has its own balance. If you give it too much energy, the healee can develop a severe headache. Do not be in a rush. You must never hurry. You must be at peace always, and give—that is, direct—a bit of energy, if you feel the need; or do not direct energy, just think of balancing.

In the past few years I have worked with many people with brain disorders. I think a lot of the mysterious illnesses of today for which we have no answer have their origin in the brain. My advice, therefore, would be to center, assess the field, and then gently move your hands over the sides of the patient's head, as well as doing whatever else has to be done. By doing Therapeutic Touch over the sides of the head you can help reestablish order in the field, and that also would be helpful to the thinking processes of the patient.

Of all the diseases I have worked with, brain diseases are the most difficult and are the most tiring. Actually, it is not the Therapeutic

Touch that is tiring. I am never tired after a healing session if I am relaxed enough, because the healing energy does not come from me, personally; I am simply directing it to go through me. What I do find taxing is trying to explain to people how they must change their lives, if they are to heal, in a way that they will do it.

Brow Chakra

The brow chakra is involved in the centering that is essential to Therapeutic Touch. It is also tied to visualization, one of the powers of the mind. In visualization, the mind—which is also associated with Therapeutic Touch healing energies, in fact with all conscious effort—can be kept still. The mind can concentrate on a picture much more easily than the emotions can, and this concentration links it to a higher level of consciousness.

In my observations of Dr. Karagulla's patients, I noticed that if a person was meditating and was good at visualization, this chakra was luminous and seemed to spread out. This suggests that visualization can have a more powerful effect than we may think possible. So I often suggest to a healee that he associate the idea of wellness or wholeness with an image such as the idea of light. In this way, the healee is making a mind picture that symbolizes his desire to get well.

Throat Chakra

When I worked with Dr. Karagulla, I saw lots of people with different diseases, including some whose thyroid had been partly removed. If there is a disease, the removal of the physical thyroid does not interfere with the chakra right away. Over time the chakra's rhythm slowly changes, but the chakra itself continues its other functions. Physically, of course, it has a lot to do with one's vitality, particularly if there is a lot of disease. It is related to the chronic fatigue syndrome, a dysfunction that can be readily perceived at this chakra site. Many people who have mental illnesses, especially those who hear sounds that are not audible to others, also have dysfunctions of the throat chakra.

Heart Chakra

Meditation and centering the consciousness automatically increase the energy of this chakra, and it becomes more luminous. If a person has heart disease—which is very common in the United States—the heart chakra will be affected. The effects can be clearly seen by one who can perceive the chakras, although they are hard to describe because the energetics are so different from what happens physically. If you can think of the chakra as resembling a system of flower petals, one of the petals may go down when there is something the matter with the heart. This is not what happens in the case of an acute heart attack, but the deteriorating condition of an ongoing disease process definitely shows up in this way. Also, the rhythm involved in the chakra's turning may be slowed down in certain sections, while it can become very fast in serious heart disease such as in those requiring an operation.

The solar plexus and the heart chakras have a profound influence on one another. However, they are often not in a harmonic relationship of movement. When they are not synchronous, that helps to produce a response of helplessness. Such a response acts as a blockage to the sense of self; then we do not feel that the strength of control is in our hands when we use the word, "I." If a patient is generating self-defeating messages such as "I cannot do anything about it," the solar plexus rhythm dominates in its expression of the difficult and the depressive. It is very hard to heal successfully in such an atmosphere.

Visualization exercises can often be very effective to harmonize the relationship of the heart and solar plexus chakras, to boost the immune system, to give a sense of the self, and to overcome a sense of hopelessness.

Solar Plexus Chakra

The solar plexus chakra is one of the most complicated centers, for it is the avenue through which our disturbed emotions get processed and then affect us physically. We often get disturbed because of our relations to others, and so do our patients. We get used to feeling a certain way and then build emotional patterns, thinking it is the only way we can feel. The power of our emotions can upset the rhythm of the solar plexus chakra, causing it to go into a state of imbalance. That in turn causes our energy to be greatly diminished.

Coordination of the Heart and Solar Plexus Chakras

In order to harness the energies of the two chakras and bring them into a more harmonious rhythm, I would think of sending energy to the heart and downward, so that the energy would go through any blockages between them. I would also ask the patient to do a visualization. This will bring in the sense of self: he is doing it. The visualization enables the patient to be an active participant in his own healing, working with you as you do Therapeutic Touch, slowly and gently.

Don't make the visualization complicated or difficult. People are not capable of a high degree of concentration if they have a great deal of pain. Let them imagine sending their pain to a distant point away from them, such as seeing it recede with an outgoing ocean tide or some other image. The important thing is that they have the sense of projecting it away from themselves; how it is done is secondary. It will give them a beginning sense of the self; the idea that they can project the images out of their system also lends a sense of control. Or you can ask patients to visualize light going through them; it will have a similar effect.

The function of the solar plexus chakra also concerns the gastrointestinal system, so people who have a lot of emotional disturbances have many gastric problems. This all is very much involved with stress, which usually extends its effects to the whole body. We can see this dynamic in people who are driven by a mental picture of being very successful. They may achieve success, but they often drain their energy in the process, seemingly using up their store of energy in early life. The adrenals become depleted, and various stomach conditions result.

You, as healer, can quiet down the entire dysfunctional process by focusing on the solar plexus chakra. If a person complains of a permanent stomachache or ulcer, I automatically think of sending energy to the solar plexus.

✆ Breathing Exercise to Quiet and ✎
Restore Solar Plexus Rhythm

When you are doing TT to quiet a patient's solar plexus, you can ask the healee to breathe consciously and rhythmically. This will help to quiet their emotions. It is the rhythm that is important, because the whole solar plexus center gets out of rhythm. If you gently do Therapeutic Touch at the same time, one act reinforces the other.

If a patient has a stomachache, you don't need to specifically think of their chakras when you give them a Therapeutic Touch treatment; you can direct your healing at the whole person or at the stomach. The chakras will work whether you think about them or not, just as our hearts work whether we think about them or not. The chakras are natural phenomena, with their own rhythm, and they are always functioning within us to keep us going, whether we are aware of them or not. What we can—and do—help is the vital-energy flow to the body's organs and other tissue.

✆ When the TT Therapist's Solar Plexus ✎
Is Negatively Affected

If you have a disturbance in your own solar plexus while doing TT, it may be a sign or warning that you are beginning to take in too much of the patient's negative energy. I suggest that you take a deep breath and stop the treatment, re-center yourself, and then go on with the healing session.

Both the heart chakra and the solar plexus are tremendously associated with emotions, but the heart chakra is much more unselfish in its orientation. The solar plexus chakra is very affected by resentment. There is an energetic difference between resentment and anger. In anger you flare up and get it off your chest; it goes out of your system, and you do not hang on to it. But people can carry resentment for many years. When you don't want to express or even acknowledge an emotion like resentment, its power is turned inward, disturbing the solar plexus chakra and thus the entire gastrointestinal tract. If a person has resentment for ten or fifteen years, that pattern will weaken the proper action of the physical organ, which will then show up in the alteration of the rhythm of the chakra.

✌️ *Visualization to Release Resentment* 👌

If you are treating a patient who is bothered by resentment relating to a particular mental image or a specific relationship, ask him to visualize the image or feeling as going through his heart, then through his solar plexus, and then out of his system. Encourage him to strongly visualize it as being literally ejected out of his vital-energy field. Hundreds of people have told me, "Dora, the one thing I can't do is visualize," so be sure to suggest something very simple. Complex visualization demands a well-developed attention span or ability to concentrate, and many people do not have that ability. In addition to making your instructions simple and clear, make sure the visualization you suggest is something about which the patient has an interest.

When you are using imagery to treat people, you do not have to talk to them very much. Remember, this is an energetic perspective we are using. Develop your TT session so that you treat slowly and gently; if something is out of kilter, you have to be very careful not to put so much energy in that you start up the pathological process.

Over and over, I must repeat: be careful about your words. Words have a powerful effect on patterns of resentment. It is important to realize that emotions and energy are very closely related in this case. You may guess the diagnosis, but be very careful about how you interpret your assessment to the patient. Under conditions of high stress, you may be one hundred percent wrong in your assessment. If you lose a patient's confidence because you use an inaccurate word, he will not receive the healing energy you are sending him to its fullest extent. In his mind, it will not reverberate with the truth.

Very few people realize the strength of our feelings, or how we build emotional patterns within ourselves based upon those feelings. When we become upset about something that is akin to our original emotional disturbance, our feelings, the psychodynamic energies, flow into that pattern. We then get emotionally upset, and our response is often greater than is warranted by the present situation. Although the current issue may not be significant in itself, its energies join the pattern of the past resentment and reinforce it, leading us to exaggerate the incident. We may flare up in disproportionate anger and, at the same time, reinforce the picture of the incident from the past. The funny thing is, we often question ourselves afterward, wondering "What is the matter with me?" In reflection, we can see that whatever happened was relatively unimportant.

If we keep in mind how resentment builds, we can curb emotional problems of this nature. When we have a strong emotional reaction, there's a direct relationship between our thinking and our feeling about it; they work together. When we get upset, there are also various physical effects: our heart begins to change rhythm, our thyroid and hormones are disturbed. At the same time, all the chakras respond to one another. They change their rhythms and therefore the state of their functioning, so there is a direct correlation between our emotional and mental states and the chakras.

Spleen Chakra

We are beginning to learn more about chronic fatigue. It is not only emotional, which means that it impacts the solar plexus chakra; it also has to do with the expending and taking in of energy. Our life-energy or *prana* comes in from the atmosphere through the spleen, from where it is distributed to the body to replenish our supply of vital-energy. People who are exhausted and have chronic fatigue syndrome are the ones who have a dysfunctional spleen chakra.

Hand and Foot Chakras

When we do Therapeutic Touch the energy goes through our hands, making the little centers in them very active. Very often when we do Therapeutic Touch, we think of the energies going out of the feet of the patient, which acts as sort of a cleansing.

Beneficial Influences
on the Chakras

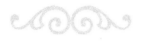

Effects of Therapeutic Touch on Therapists' Chakras

IF YOU DO A LOT OF THERAPEUTIC TOUCH, your chakras come into a brighter, more radiant, functioning. The chakras that are the most affected by giving Therapeutic Touch are the heart chakra—since you are going out in compassion—and the brow and crown chakras. The involvement of the brow and the crown chakras comes with the conscious sense of direction or intentionality. The consciousness of those chakras and the directive force of your brain are operating together when you say, "I am dealing with heart disease, and I am sending energy toward the heart."

Those whom I have known for ten or twenty years who have been practicing Therapeutic Touch do not realize how much they have changed. Giving treatments has automatically speeded up their chakras. They have also developed a finer sensitivity to their intuition. As a result of working together harmoniously in teams, they do not take everything that happens so personally. They connect to their inner self and their expanded worldview brings a spiritual perspective and a higher level of energies into their being. This helps them change and makes them more effective healers than when they began. Even the well-known healers I have met in my life have appeared to change a great deal over time, because through the process of healing, they too became more empathetic in their understanding and their perceptions.

In Therapeutic Touch the therapists have a chance to project their energy for helpful purposes. This has given meaning to their lives, which have changed greatly in many cases. I think this has brought them self-confidence. They report that they have become more psychologically grounded and centered, more mindful, more intuitive, and more trusting of their intuition. They have a resolute intentionality and a better perspective on their relationships to people in pain. They are able to maintain their center of quiet and project that stillness for the benefit of those in need.

When a Therapeutic Touch therapist is centered and contributing goodwill, she is also physically strengthened. She has access to a new source of energy so that she can keep going. When she is working in a hospital setting, she does not think in terms of all the pain. She thinks, "What can I do to help?" As a nurse, she may have already been doing all she could physically for her patients; now she can also say, "I am giving you a little energy and peace," which I think contributes to everyone involved. Therapeutic Touch develops a sense of giving at a different level, and that lifts one's own energy a great deal, making the whole thing worthwhile, on many fronts. Life becomes deeply satisfying and meaningful.

⟲ Meditation on the Heart Chakra ⟳

Some people meditate on their own chakras from top down. I would not do it that way. I would start with the heart. When I go out and help with healing, it is my heart chakra that is expanding. Meditating on the heart chakra will help you and will probably have a beneficial effect on others as well, because the energy of love is spontaneous and reactive to everything in its sphere of influence. This is the easiest way to reach a person when doing TT, for the energy of the heart chakra is genuine. You can feel it as it goes out to the person. By consciously directing an outward flow of love to a person, you may speed up his or her ability to have a first inkling of the unity of the inner self.

Bringing the functions of the heart chakra into your daily life in this way also offers you a wonderful opportunity to develop a clear recognition of the differences between sympathy and compassion, and to further develop compassion. Compassion, in my language, is the feeling and understanding—and I stress this—that each person has within himself this inner self and that we are bound together at that level of consciousness.

Therapeutic Touch and Auras

A person's aura is their emotional energy manifesting around—actually interpenetrating—the body. Sending goodwill and energy for the healing of a disease positively affects the aura of both therapist and patient. This is basic to the Therapeutic Touch process. The moment a person gets upset, those feelings are at once distributed in their aura. If the energy is intense it affects the chakras. A Therapeutic Touch treatment changes the color and subtle energy patterns of the patient's aura as the patient lessens and then loses his anxiety. The therapist projects quieting colors and by so doing helps to make a change, and most people feel very much quieter. You can affect an aura very quickly; most people rapidly feel revitalized. They also readily feel the goodwill, which some of them need so much. They feel so lonely, and it gives them a sense that somebody really cares.

Therapist's Effect on the Patient's Chakras

The Therapeutic Touch process tries to alter physical dysfunction; it does not try to effect a change in the chakras. However, a TT therapist *can, and does, alter the energy flow in the body*. I reiterate this because it is an important distinction to understand. When the therapist picks up something that is disturbing around a patient's stomach, she often thinks that she is picking up something regarding the chakra. Well, I believe in that, but I do not think that is what she is going to alter by her healing. I think we make a big mistake if we try to tune into each chakra when we do Therapeutic Touch. It is nonsense, for they are related to each other and usually work in unison.

The chakras may not be functioning properly when disease is present in the body. The only way you can affect the chakras is if you can get in touch with their rhythm, which will give you the sense of a disease or not-disease state. Affecting the energy of the chakras takes concentration; you have to be very calm within yourself first. Then you can send thoughts of peace and help to give the chakras energy flow. If you are treating heart disease or an emotional upset, for instance, you can be helpful by sending thoughts of energy with your intentionality, giving the chakras a little more energy to balance the situation. You may feel a disturbance near the heart, a cue of heat or cold, but that does not mean you have picked up the chakra. You have felt the effects of whatever is wrong with the heart. When you quiet a person and their heart becomes calm, the heart chakra will follow suit.

If a patient is in overwhelming pain, he or she loses a sense of the "I," the individual self. You can, by Therapeutic Touch, restore the sense of self by first relaxing the patient. Then you can send them energy. In doing that, you will help the chakras to harmonize. The bodily process is very important. We always want to separate the body from the consciousness, but the two actually work together incessantly. They are never separated, unless a person is unconscious.

When you finish assessing during a TT treatment, it is very important that you think for a moment that you are going out to help that person as a whole. The first thing you do is send that idea of wholeness, which you could translate in physical terms as coordinated functioning. Then your visualization will be more realistic and the energies you project will function together in an integrated fashion. The body and the consciousness of the patient will distribute the energy where it is needed.

The energy will first go toward that person at the physical energy level. Then your sense of calmness will reach them at the emotional and mental levels. If you can do that for them, you bring back in a very small way their sense that *there is a self*; then they can think, "I am going to get better." So you bring back their sense that there is more to consciousness than just the emotions and the physical body. Slowly, when they get better, they will reconnect to all their levels of consciousness.

You are not trying to convince the healee. You are trying to help him function to his potential as a human being. That is the prime purpose of healing. If you can make him interested, then coming to a place like Pumpkin Hollow where we do so many TT sessions can change his worldview. But if a person is in tremendous pain, I am not going to think about changing his worldview; I will work to lessen his pain. A change in worldview will come when his sense of self comes in more consciously.

I am often asked how important it is for people learning about Therapeutic Touch to learn about the chakras. I do not know about the importance. If you are interested, you can learn something about the mechanism. But in the healing, you cannot just put your hand on someone and say, "You're cured," or "The chakra is cured." That is imagination. It has to be something the patient experiences and not what is said to occur. He does not have to experience it in terms of chakras. He is experiencing it in terms of his consciousness. And when he experiences it in terms of consciousness, his chakras will change.

The degree of healing depends upon the strength and clarity of your intentionality—your clear, focused thinking. Just feeling kind is not the same thing as having intentionality. I think that intentionality develops your intuition. When you use your hands to send the healing energy, your intention is pouring out toward a previously determined goal. As you use your heart chakra to add healing energies, a powerful relationship occurs between the heart and the hands.

If you do Therapeutic Touch with a deep intent, and you are in harmony, you can send energy in a very positive way. If you really make a relationship with the patient, he has to be able to accept it unconsciously. Once you have formed a relationship and he responds, he has to act. People have to alter their chakras for themselves. The individual response of the person is crucial. I must stress that it deals with consciousness. Your standing in front of the patient and moving your hands is not going to make too much difference, but you can have an effect if you can get the person's consciousness to cooperate with you. To do that you must listen to it, very carefully.

When you relate to the patient's inner self, you are not relating to something outside of you. It is what you quietly think in your mind. It is not your hands; it is your consciousness. The moment you get to the sense of the inner self, you reach an altogether different level of consciousness. If you can help a patient to do that for himself, that is healing. Even a glimpse of it, a momentary response, opens, not the chakra, but the relationship between his inner self and his chakras, and you have affected that.

Patients themselves can work on their own chakras, to a certain extent. If they are able to relax very deeply and think of energy coming into their body, it is possible for them to stimulate their own energy to an appreciable level. The first thing they must do is deeply relax; that is paramount. Then, if the condition permits it, deep abdominal breathing would help stimulate the intake of fresh energy. Moderate meditative practices will help, too. Visualizing energy going through the entire body can be very effective, particularly if the healee can lie out in the sunshine for a short while. Visualizing appropriate colors permeating the body can also be helpful. In reference to nutrition, if one is very depleted and if there is difficulty with the solar plexus chakra, it can be helpful to drink and eat in small quantities at a time and to do this more often than is the usual case; this may help to speed up the recovery of the chakras.

✍ Bringing Harmony to the Chakra System ✍

One way to develop the chakras so they will evenly work together is trying to be as harmonious, or integrated, in your behaviors as possible. If you get constantly upset and your emotions are out of balance, you may function adequately for some time, but you will not experience harmony in the chakra system as a whole. It is we, ourselves, who can produce this harmony or integration. Nobody else can do it for us. It is like exercising a muscle; you, yourself, must support the coordination of the chakra system by your actions.

Effects of Meditation on the Chakras

In meditation, particularly, we feel we have a level of consciousness that is somehow connected with the inner self and its insights. The information conveyed is accompanied by a strong sense of certainty and profundity, taking it beyond the realm of ordinary intuition. It is what we might call a true experience of interiority.

When a person is meditating, the crown, the brow, and the heart chakras are tremendously affected by one another. Meditation enhances the harmony of these three chakras, but they are each also functioning on their own. Meditation quiets a person. Feeling the positive emotions of love is also part of meditation, for the heart is the center for a person in deep meditation. In a person who meditates I can see a greater shine or radiance at the core of their heart chakra, as well as a greater expansion of the chakra. The heart chakra is also very important in the considered use of consciousness. When a person is thinking creatively, getting new ideas, the heart, brow, and crown chakras also work closely together: with deep thinking and visualization, intuition arises spontaneously.

When we do Therapeutic Touch, we very often get an insight about what the patient is feeling or experiencing at that moment. We cannot count upon having such flashes of insight, but they do come, indicating that the brow chakra is working in harmony with the heart chakra. We not only have the intuition; the mental level of our consciousness is also partly involved. The whole brain is affected, particularly the pituitary, because it is an understanding as well as a perception.

When a person is tremendously disturbed, I can see that there is a disrupted pattern in their chakras. If TT is then done on that person or they meditate, the rhythm of the pattern can be changed. I have seen people who are very emotionally disturbed get an insight through meditation and significantly change: their aura and the rhythm of the affected chakra is changed. Once the rhythm changes in one chakra, it slowly affects the rhythm in all.

If you could get somebody who is disturbed to meditate voluntarily—to meditate for even one minute to start with—he will have made the first step toward a change. If he really wants change, I think his inner self will come down and help. Doing something routinely will slowly break up the patterns of dysrhythmia that characterize the chakras of many people who are very sick. Most people who are disturbed do not want to do something regularly, so start with encouraging them to do something very simple. You have to help them relate to their difficulties and also give them a visualization that suits their particular state of mind. If they can mentally experience that they have achieved a time of being peaceful, of being more like the self they would like to be, it might give them the impetus to change. But *they* must do it.

CLINICAL APPLICATIONS OF THERAPEUTIC TOUCH

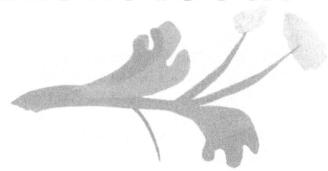

Introductory Comments

The sensitivity of the Therapeutic Touch therapist improves as a consequence of persevering at the practice of the assessment, fostering her awareness of the finer levels of consciousness of the healee. As all the levels of consciousness interpenetrate, the heightened sensitivity of the TT therapist enables her to become aware of the "whole person" who is the healee. She perceives a sense of his totality during the assessment or during the reassessment at the end of the session when the TT process has made her awareness more acute. With this increased sensitivity, the therapist very frequently gains a sharper insight into what it is about the healee that is out of balance, and she may have an intuition about the cause of the problem as well. The progression is not additive, but it is multifactored. It happens unobtrusively and—most frequently—very quickly.

In the TT practice of sustained centering the therapist focuses her attention on her heart chakra, where she becomes aware of a sense of profound peace and stillness. Over time she begins to realize that these signs of inner quietude are symbolic signals of her connection to the inner self. Upon that recognition, she allows that sense of stillness to pervade her fields of consciousness, and she uses those gentle, tranquil handmaidens of order as the medium through which she projects healing energies to the healee. Once she can maintain that state of consciousness for even a short while—two minutes, as Dora recommends, is a good rule of thumb in the beginning—she can permit it to touch her life, allowing it to become conscious in her acts of daily living. Then her field of consciousness gets into the "habit" and she may find, as many others have, that it enables her to transmit a sense of stability, equanimity, and even a hint of grace and presence to others who are in fear, confusion, or inner turmoil.

Such an ability is particularly helpful when a person is working with frightened children, people in panic, many psychotics, particularly those who are schizophrenic, and also persons who are in final transition. One gets the sense that it is the inner self at work, and it is working with the unstable person at a profound transverbal level, inner self to inner self. As a result of such experiences an underlying spiritual quality makes itself known to the therapist while she is working with the Therapeutic Touch process.

Dora makes a point of suggesting ways of overcoming base emotions, such as fear, anger, and resentment, because their effect on the fields of consciousness is that of blocking the fine energy pathways the inner self engages to act through the life activities of the therapist.

As noted in the introductory comments to Section III, certain bodily systems are more sensitive to the TT process than are others. One of these is the genitourinary system in both males and females. However, only certain organs of the endocrine system demonstrate that sensitivity. The adrenal glands, physiologically located on the top of the kidneys, are extremely sensitive to Therapeutic Touch. In fact, when a TT therapist— even one who is a novice—passes her hand chakra through the vital-energy field overlying the adrenals of a healee who is very depleted of prana, she will feel a decided shift in subtle energy flow. The adrenals seem to "slurp" up the prana flowing from the therapist's hand chakras. It is not unusual that very rapidly thereafter the healee will report a sense of increased vitality. In fact this can be so reliably done to increase the energy level of the healee that a tried and true assertion of those who teach Therapeutic Touch is, ". . . if you don't pick up any significant cues during the TT assessment, give energy to the area of the adrenals anyway. It will only be helpful to the healee, even if you do not understand why."

At this time we do not know just why this happens so invariably and so rapidly. As a rationale one thinks of the quickening effects of epinephrine—the major hormone secreted by the adrenals—on the musculature and the circulatory systems of the body. Although over forty doctoral dissertations, more than twenty postdoctoral researches, and innumerable clinical studies on Therapeutic Touch have been completed at this writing, no one has tackled this interesting question on these expeditious and effective clinical correlates of the Therapeutic Touch process.

One of the major effects of epinephrine is on blood pressure, and one of the highly reliable effects of Therapeutic Touch is the reduction of high blood pressure readings. Interestingly, this is done using the visualization of "the healing blue," generally thought of as royal blue, while doing Therapeutic Touch with a person who has high blood pressure. The protocol for doing this was developed by Dora and me during the early days of TT, when we were trying to determine the parameters of the Therapeutic Touch process. We did a series of pilot studies on the effect of TT on hypertension, using as experimental subjects a convenient sample of a dozen women between the ages of sixty and seventy-five years who had been medically diagnosed as being hypertensive. All of these women demonstrated a diastolic reading (the bottom number of the blood pressure ratio) of over 100 and a systolic reading of over 200, each person acting as her own control in a simple pre-post design. The study period was for five consecutive days, with each healee receiving one TT session each day. After having her blood pressure taken and recorded by a nurse who was not otherwise involved in the study, each subject was given Therapeutic Touch by a TT therapist for twenty to twenty-five minutes. During this time the TT therapist visualized the healing blue color permeating through the healee while she did Therapeutic Touch. At the end of the TT session, the blood pressure reading of the healee was again recorded. The healee rested for about ten minutes post-treatment and then returned home. Healees continued whatever medication and dietary regime they had been on previous to the study.

The results occurred more quickly and were sustained longer than we had anticipated. After one session, the systolic readings were under 200 for all healees. They ranged from 178 to 150, with an average systolic of 164. The diastolic readings were all under 100, ranging from 90 to 72, with an average diastolic reading of 80. The readings were maintained at that level throughout the five days of the study. We repeated the study, with similar results, and since then many others have replicated our study so that the findings have attained an impressive reliability. It is because of this reliability that the use of the projection of color in appropriate instances has become a part of standard Therapeutic Touch treatment.

As was mentioned, the findings of this study exceeded our expectations. While Dora could directly perceive the effects of the projection of color on the vital-energy and psychodynamic fields, I had to perceive this—and other ways of using subtle energies that we later included in the TT process—in ways that were very different from Dora's incredible abilities. Luckily for me, I have a good intuition. As I learned ways of studying it to learn how to gauge its reliability, it helped my understanding of the TT process considerably. However, my learning about the healing properties of color and how to use them during the healing interaction was more pragmatic.

One day, while giving a talk on healing in a cathedral, I noticed sunlight playing through the old stained glass windows and bathing the congregation in various colors of light. The thought occurred to me that I might be able to experience the effect of the different colors by sitting in the tinted light of the beams. Intrigued with the idea, I returned and spent over an hour one afternoon sitting in various pews, centering my consciousness, and then being mindful of any changes in consciousness that occurred. The result was very interesting: I could detect a distinct, though subtle, change in mood as I experienced the differently colored light beams. The shaft of colored light that had the most pronounced effect was the blue that beamed through the stained glass depicting the Virgin Mary. The next most effective shaft of colored light was yellow, but I felt it differently. Whereas the blue was soothing, comforting, relaxing, even tranquilizing in its effect, the yellow light was more arousing, invigorating, and stimulating. I carried on these studies of colored light for some months and I found that I could replicate in my mind the colors instilled in me when I was in the cathedral, even when I was not in the glow of the light. I also found that I could visualize these colors and project them to a healee during TT sessions for specific effects. I discussed these findings with Dora, Dora continued her own studies of color, and the use of color in our TT sessions quickly caught on (see Krieger, *Accepting Your Power to Heal*, p. 60, for more on our explorations regarding the use of color visualization in TT).

We have been very effective in using the healing blue to calm, sedate, or slow down imbalanced subtle energies. The blue that was chosen was that of the light that filtered down through the stained glass representation of the robes of the Virgin Mary. This particular blue was so effective that it aroused my interest in tracing its use. With the help of a friend who was an artist, we found that it has been associated with the Virgin Mary, or the Mother of the World, since earliest times, and that the tradition was perpetuated through the medieval art guilds to modern times.

Besides blue and yellow, we have added the visualization and projection of light green, rose, violet, orange, and clear light to our TT repertoire (see Krieger, *Therapeutic Touch Inner Workbook*, p. 130, for a more detailed account of the situations for which these colors are used). We have found that it is not the projection of the colors themselves that makes a significant difference in the vital-energy flow, but that visualizing colors helps the way the therapist thinks or evokes a particular psychological mood.

Dora encouraged personal experimentation. She gave us the freedom to think deeply and to imagine freely, but she expected of her students the same self-discipline she demanded of herself and, therefore, she held the line at sheer fantasy, uncontrolled emotional outbursts, or blatant exaggeration. However, she had an incredible and contagious sense of humor that saw both her patients and her students through many difficult situations.

One result of this casual environment had amusing consequences. It concerns a very simple way we had of naming TT techniques as we developed them. When we passed our hands through a healee's vital-energy field during an assessment, we could feel sensations that felt like heat or cold. Often as we worked with the healee, the sensations of heat would increase. That gave rise to the use of the saying "He's cooked!" to describe a healee who has had enough projection of healing energies. Under certain conditions, a vital-energy field that is in a state of imbalance feels rough, as though it has uneven, wavy ruffles. So when we cleared a healee's field of that condition, we called it "unruffling."

Several early students experimented with the projection of various colors. One of our findings was that it was possible to teach oneself to hold more than one color in mind at the same time and project that combination to the healee. This led Mikey—then a mere medical resident, but now a distinguished specialist in emergency pediatric medicine—to exercise both his fine sensibilities and a roguish sense of humor to come up with a novel classification, "Think plaid!" So, besides the ordinary strangenesses that TT therapists are heir to, we "think plaid," find "ruffles" in the seemingly empty space around people, and we "cook" our patients!

The Context of Wholeness

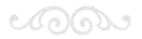

I WANT TO BEGIN BY REMINDING YOU that centering—the conscious withdrawal of your focus to your heart—is at the core of Therapeutic Touch. It is here that you can become consciously aware of the peace and stillness that characterize the link with the inner self. If, even for a few minutes daily, you can draw upon this and identify with that peace and quiet, you will be opening yourself to the source of your healing energy to a greater degree, without being distracted by undisciplined feelings. Then whatever you become aware of—Therapeutic Touch, your activities of daily life—will be filtered through a concentrated atmosphere of peace and stillness. You will also project that peace and healing to your patients.

It is more important for you to center your consciousness when you are preparing to heal than to tell patients, "I love you," and hug them. The patients are disturbed; they have pain; they do not know their future; and they are afraid. If we discipline ourselves—and it is a discipline—our first desire should not be to hug them, however sorry we feel, but to help them reduce their anxiety. We want to help them forget their close identity with their illness for the few minutes of the Therapeutic Touch interaction. First give them the energy to quiet themselves. If you send out a sense of peace, they will relax in your hands. Then, if you know how, help to reduce their pain.

Several studies have been done in hospitals, and they all conclude that patients who receive Therapeutic Touch pre-operatively are in the hospital a shorter time. This result is attributed to the rapid relaxation response that occurs during TT and is then sustained. If you can center and project an atmosphere in which a patient can relax deeply, you are doing something significant to help.

That is why it is so important that you are relaxed while doing Therapeutic Touch. If you are uptight because you want to help or you want to succeed, you do something to yourself that is not really compatible with healing. When you get tense like that, you are unconsciously thinking more about your own reactions to the healing than focusing on the patient's needs. During the healing interaction you have in front of you another person who is sick and vulnerable. As a healer you are the transmitter of healing energy, to enable that person's health. It is basic, therefore, that you center and forget about yourself for the time being in the interest of meeting the needs of the patient; that is the charge you accepted in doing Therapeutic Touch.

When you are projecting healing energy and thinking of it flowing, you need to think of it going to the totality of the person. You are really trying to have a relationship with the inner self of the patient in order to effect an impersonal and caring transmission of healing power. After centering, and before healing, you want to reach in to your own inner self and then "out" to the inner self of the patient; then do whatever has to be done to help that person.

I unconsciously reach out to the inner self—the "whole person"—when I do Therapeutic Touch. If you find the concept of the "whole person" difficult, you can think instead of bringing order into the system. Remember that if a person is sick, part of his system is not functioning in a coordinated manner, so the energy flows themselves are dysfunctional. What is important is that all the functions of the whole body work together in harmony. In your assessment you may not have picked up some necessary information. However, if you keep your mind on the wholeness of the healee, his body will pick up, in an integrated fashion, whatever it needs as a totality.

It is this context of wholeness that allows TT to work in such a wide variety of illnesses. When your mind is involved with the conceptualization of wholeness, your energies are outgoing. Even in cases of deep depression or near-panic anxieties in the healee, you will not be taking in those energies. You may have an image or a sense of the sadness or other distresses of the healee, but you do not take in his emotions, because you are sending out energies at the same time. Of course, critical to all of this is that you start out in a centered state of consciousness and maintain that state throughout the session.

When we project energy in Therapeutic Touch what we are basically doing is giving the patient's body access to enough vital-energy to fight the disease process itself. The body, through its immune system, has to be strong enough to do that. With the immune system working overtime during an illness, often the energy levels of the patient do not have the capacity to regenerate sufficiently. If the person's mind and physical body are well integrated, he can deal with his own problems. However, if the energy is greatly depleted and there is tremendous fear, the fear further reduces the strength of the immune system, keeping the system down longer. Although the inner self is always there for the individual, it does get blocked by the fear. This blocking does not occur in people who act in a more integrated manner, enabling them to pass on peacefully when they die.

We should consider this when we are engaged in the healing process. Even if the Therapeutic Touch therapist cannot do much for a critically ill person, helping the patient to relax will ease their passage from this world to that other one. You should not feel discouraged if the symptoms are not reduced; this is another aspect of healing in which you can still be helpful. You can help a person not only with physical death, but also with the spiritual aspects of his experience.

You can also do healing at a distance, for persons going for surgery. Many patients facing surgery feel very insecure, wondering if it will be the last time they will see those they love. They need to be sent a sense of security and caring. If they know that you are meditating on them, it often makes them feel very safe.

When I do healing, I try to be still and to have a sense of nonattachment to the results; I will do the best that I can for the person in need, meanwhile fully recognizing that the results—good or bad—are not totally in my hands. Even though we always want to be successful, we cannot be, because no person's destiny is fully in our hands. If you are dealing with many people in your Therapeutic Touch practice, some of them will not respond; you have to accept that. People who have not accepted that sometimes feel that they are to blame, which blocks the flow of healing energy. We also have to accept that we are human beings, and that some days we don't do so well.

Different people, without any doubt, react differently, and at first some people will reject the support you offer. Remember that a person who thinks of himself as being sick has built a mind-picture at that level of consciousness. The pictures that are built up are usually very firmly embedded and sometimes can severely block a person's receptivity to the healing energy. Somehow you have to help the patient to break through that fixed idea, *to repattern that flow*. If you truly relax him and encourage him, he can break that link. Once he feels better and feels he can express himself in some way, those pictures of himself can break up completely. It will not happen immediately, but it *can* happen. That will be a beginning of real healing and an indication that the patient is accepting the healing energy. Although very few people completely reject that energy, many are hesitant and uncertain. However, they will usually open to the healing once they experience a sense of peace.

Intentionality and Healing

The understanding of intentionality makes a great difference in how you use your energy during healing. I have noticed that many people—even after some time of practicing Therapeutic Touch—don't focus on their hand chakras or think very clearly while they center. They think vaguely of the energy and the body. You need to put the full force of your mind on the fact that you are sending a healing energy, a finely ordered system. The intentionality of thinking of the person as whole, in his totality as a human being, is of core importance.

I am able to understand why a person is in pain because I can see what is blocking the energy flow. That kind of perception is not necessary, however, to become aware of pain in the TT assessment. After I perceive the problem, I have the intentionality to project specific energies to that site, and it does have an effect. With some of our patients, with end-stage cancer, for example, Therapeutic Touch enables them to breathe without pain, and they feel better. But it takes *informed intentionality* to accomplish this, not just going through the motions of healing techniques or the simple sending of goodwill to the healee. If you have informed intentionality, you can see the effect directly, for the patients improve.

e⁄⁄@ *Using Intentionality During* *@⁄⁄*
the Healing Process

As always, begin with relaxing the patient to give him a respite from
concern about his disease. If you then think of sending the energy,
the patient's relaxed body will absorb it more readily. You can even
say to the patient, "Don't think about your illness now. For this short
while, just relax completely." While you are relaxing the patient, that
is also the beginning for you, for initiating your concentration to get
the energy flowing. You also need to relax and feel the flow as it grad-
ually comes through you. Then focus your mind very strongly for a
few minutes upon an energy flow going through the area of illness.
That will keep your own mind in closer contact with the healing
process. Do not think of the pain. Keep your attention focused on a
harmonic order being restored within that person's energy systems.
Even though nobody actually knows exactly where the healing
energy will go, it will flow in an orderly way through the patient's
body, given the opportunity.

Specific Applications of the "Whole Person" Concept

Although the concept of the "whole person" seems to have practically
no meaning for most people, TT adds that perspective. Let us take multiple sclerosis as an example. There is an orderly process going on—life
itself—but myelinating disease is a deteriorating pattern that affects the
person's walking. Part of the disease process brings in an anxiety also,
because the person never knows what he or she can do from day to day,
and this reinforces a sense of impending disaster. With TT we can help
support the orderly flow. We can also help the person accept the day by
day variations, without dwelling on them. People who are sick want to
dwell on their disease, but we can help them to resist that and to go on.

ⅇ⁄ᵒ   Working with Persons Who   ᵒᐯᵔ
Have Multiple Sclerosis

When I work with these persons, first of all I send them extra energy so that they can function more normally, with a sense of well-being and the energy to face what must be done. Then I combine that with a sense of wholeness—of the inner self—and that helps them to be calmer. I talk to them about the simplest of things, and I think of them as being able to deal with their emotions about not being able to function. I help them recognize that it is not their fault, for they often look upon themselves as partial failures. I can help them a lot more if I can see them a few times. When they are not in pain I give them exercises, too, to build what function they have. That also helps to build their self-confidence.

Often when one concentrates only on the surface, the healing process does not interact with the deeper aspects of the person. This is especially true in reference to problems of the circulatory system. I have learned to begin TT by working on the back of the patient's neck because the tension the patient is under makes something queer happen to the usual energy flows. Quietly directing energy to the base of the neck helps calm the patient's fears.

From my experience the kidneys are even more important than the heart. They are very often involved in disease processes and in physiological dysfunctions, so it is not always easy to assess whether there is something wrong with the kidneys themselves. The kidney function often slows down for various other reasons, such as something the healee has eaten, or an emotional upset. And, in some cases, the kidneys may be prone to future illnesses. Although they may not necessarily be diseased, they perform such a central function in the well being of the body that I always send them energy whenever I notice any cue in that area of the body.

Balancing the Energies of Persons with Heart Problems

Once the person is in a relaxed state of mind, think quietly of the healing energy going through your own energy fields. Then direct it through the top of the patient's head and toward the place in the heart area where you first picked up the cue. Then unruffle the vital-energy field by placing your hand chakras close to the healee's body (with palms facing away from the body) and gently but firmly moving your hands outward. Your hand chakras will feel "full," as though they were carrying the chaotic or congested energy away from the body. At the end of the arc outward, let that energy go, to dissipate into the surrounding atmosphere. Then, direct the energies to the legs and out the feet chakras. Repeat the entire procedure slowly and gently three or four times and then let the patient rest. This strategy can be repeated after several minutes if there still is need; however, do it gently and rhythmically. Under no circumstances do TT for an excessive period of time.

Techniques for Pain
Reduction

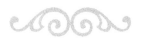

PAIN IS ONE OF THE MOST DIFFICULT SYMPTOMS to handle and many questions arise about it: How can we deal with pain? How can TT help those in pain? Do some people experience more pain than others; is the degree of pain felt dependent on the nervous system and the affect of the individual? Do people go through comparable experiences but not register the same degree of pain? Does temperament have anything to do with it?

Some people apparently do experience more pain than others. Perhaps temperament has something to do with it, but basically it is the nervous system that one inherits and its consequent sensitivity that is crucial in a person's response to pain. There also is a strong cultural component to how one regards pain, as well as an evident relation between one's social class and how pain is regarded. In many parts of the world, among the very poor, people are trained from the time they are children to endure pain. Then there are the sensitive, often high-strung, people who can endure pain, if they make up their minds, but who cannot if they do not discipline themselves. People who are sensitive often have to cope with a strong mental picture of the pain.

Pain can originate at any of the levels of consciousness and, therefore, it has a very large spectrum of intensities and is an indication of many symptoms. It can accompany almost all physical disorders and can be generated by both emotional and mental distress as well as by spiritual anguish. Over the years, it has been demonstrated that Therapeutic Touch can alleviate or abolish a wide variety of painful symptoms. Consequently, I have provided both general as well as specific suggestions for the treatment of pain with TT.

༄ᩘ᩠   Using Therapeutic Touch to Treat Pain   ᩤᩘ᩠

At first, forget completely about controlling the pain. Begin, as always, by relaxing the tension in the shoulders. While it is not easy, you can relax a person in pain with Therapeutic Touch by completely surrounding and permeating him in a visualization of royal blue for a few minutes. That will help to quiet down his whole nervous system. When you feel he has quieted down, even a little bit, then work on the pain. You will find that he will respond much better.

When you are beginning to treat the pain, start by putting your hand directly above the patient's head, palm down, above the pain center, the thalamus, in the middle of the brain. Keeping your hand above the head, begin sending blue very gently for a short time. Distribute that energy through his shoulders, and then throughout the patient's body. Keep in mind the patient as a whole person, a total being, and send the blue through his heart center outward toward the periphery.

Remember that patients often have mental pictures of being ill and in pain that slow down the effect of Therapeutic Touch. If they feel relaxed and secure they are more likely to let go of that mental picture. If you know the patient, ask him to think of someone or something he loves, even if it is a cat, a dog, or a tree, while you are focusing on his heart center. Keep the visualization simple, for a person in pain has difficulty maintaining focus. Doing TT while he visualizes something pleasant like that can help dissipate his attachment to a mental picture of himself as being so ill. It is not an easy thing to do, but TT can relax him, and that gives you access.

Then send that energy to the solar plexus, which is often a center of disturbance, particularly when there is strong pain. Even if it is not the center of the disease, many people get digestive upsets from the stress of the pain, as well as from anxiety and other emotional problems that lodge in the solar plexus. After the pain is over, you can again treat the solar plexus by sending it the blue. That will reinforce the relaxation and the relief will last longer.

After directing the energy down through the legs and feet, go once more to the shoulders and try to reinforce the relaxation.

It is important to know that the area at the back of the neck is often where tension and pain will be picked up in the assessment. The area at the base of the skull connects directly to the brain, where our sense of pain is primarily located. So you may be tapping into the pain center rather than into the site of the disease. This is particularly important to remember when two therapists are working on a healee during the assessment. The person working on the front of the healee is usually seeking out patterns of energy or evaluating the quality of energy flow or checking on a sense of imbalance over an organ. In all of this, she is trying to connect with the person in the back, integrating her efforts so to be in harmony with that person as they work together. A difficulty may arise if the therapist in the back thinks very much about the spine. Then the healee may experience a lot of tension focused in the back of the neck, between the shoulders.

In a way, pain stimulates a person, so constant pain is very exhausting. We have seen, particularly in hospices, that there are persons for whom narcotics, even morphine, will not take away the pain. To help them, you want to focus on quieting and dulling the pain. Pain is at the level of body-consciousness. However, interwoven with that are certain aspects of the level of consciousness that has to do with the emotions. If you use royal blue, it will work on the patient's emotions as well as sedating the tissues physiologically.

ஆ   *Using TT for Intractable Pain*   ௸

First go straight to the pain center in the middle of the brain and flood it with visualized royal blue. Then project a stream of blue through the body while you think of it as dulling the excitability of the pain. If you are working on an adult who has been on narcotics for a long while, spend more time on the head in a gentle way; do not exert much effort. Although many narcotics lower the respiratory rate, using blue while treating sedated patients will not injure them. After a few minutes, project the energy we call "green," thinking of the color of green grass going through the person and helping him to feel peaceful. In other words, you are sending him energy as you end the session. The green will work to balance him, lift his spirits, and help him to sleep more normally.

Specific Pain Treatments

✐ TT for Persons with Chronic Back Pain ๑๖

Chronic back pain is one of the hardest problems to deal with, both in traditional medicine and in TT. The spine is moving all the time, and that adds to the pain. The back is very difficult to work with, especially when the person has had several operations before you see them. However, I think you can reduce the pain. First of all, I would spend a lot of time high on the back of the neck, in the area right under the skull. Then work down the spine, visualizing a great deal of royal blue in the center of the lower spine, at the curvature, but doing TT fairly slowly down the entirety of the spine. Repeat this several times. In this case, you can use all the energy you are able to transmit to the patient; you do not have to be delicate about it.

✐ TT for Persons with Arthritis ๑๖

People who have arthritis have great difficulty in walking, and the problem is most often concentrated in the knees and the hipbones. However, when doing TT to the knees, place your hands behind the kneecaps rather than over them. The healing process will occur more rapidly that way, and its effects will last for a longer time.

✐ TT for Burn Patients ๑๖

Several TT therapists have successfully worked with patients with severe burns, bringing about a very rapid reduction or disappearance of pain. The important thing to keep in mind while treating persons with burns is to visualize the healing blue penetrating deeply into the skin. Remember to include the solar plexus area; you will have to work a little longer on it than is usual with other ailments. I think you will find that it will take about five minutes or so before the patient will feel relief.

✑◎   *TT for Patients with Leg Cramps* ◎⤳

I have not treated many patients with claudication, also called reflex sympathetic dystrophy, but I recommend doing it in two stages. It is always good to start with the head, over the area of the thalamus. Then—when you begin to work in the shoulder area to reinforce the relaxation response—direct the energy straight to the legs, going through the knees on the way to and through the feet. Then send a lot of royal blue to the solar plexus and, again, focus very strongly on the knees. The knee controls a lot of the healing energy going down the body; it is like an energizing focus point that affects the whole leg. I would then work separately with each foot. But, again, first think about energy going through the whole body to the feet. While you are working, go back to treating the whole body two or three times and then go to the feet again.

✑◎   *TT for Mothers in Labor* ◎⤳

Be sure to center yourself before going into an active labor and delivery room, because the energy in the room itself may seem to be very chaotic.

When mothers are in labor, our "standard" healing royal blue works very well to reduce their pain. Remember, however, that the mother also needs energy. It is tremendously hard work to deliver a baby and the continual pain over long periods of time can be exhausting. The technique here concentrates on the rebalancing of the whole field. So I suggest that you visualize a light blue color; under no condition use the darker shades of blue. Give her energy, and the balancing will also help in energizing her whenever she needs it.

✑◎   *TT for Babies in Pain* ◎⤳

The basic thing to keep in mind when treating babies is that they are very sensitive and respond more quickly than adults. Move your hands very slowly and do not put too much energy into Therapeutic Touch treatments with them. If you give them too much energy, it will irritate them. They will get something like a headache, and cry about that, not about the original pain. Think of the solar plexus, too, in treating them, because quite a lot of babies have pain in the abdomen.

I understand that there are newborn babies who actually become irritated when the healing blue is used, but that a pale sky-blue seems to work well, if it is used very gently. Some TT therapists have tried sending gentle puffs of sky-blue energy from the baby's head to its feet. It is very good if you do that; in fact, whatever color you use while treating a baby should be of a light hue.

Using TT for Pain of Drug Withdrawal

Drug withdrawal also can be painful. Such patients' nerves have been dulled, the drugs having made the person oblivious to pain. When the drug is discontinued, the nerves have no support to dampen the pain. The patient feels the full brunt of the pain and is usually very tired as well. Project the energy of grass green, thinking of it as penetrating deeply and flooding the nervous system. The green will feed and stimulate the person's jangled and overstressed nerves. The person may feel the effect reasonably quickly if the energy penetrates deeply.

Using TT with Newborn Babies of Drug Addicted Mothers

Babies who have absorbed drugs from their addicted mothers in utero must be weaned away from the effect of the drugs, and the withdrawal is painful. To ease their pain, project energies corresponding to a very light green, because the newborns need energy. Send these energies very gently, very lightly about the sides of the head, keeping your hands moving quietly all the time. Do not actually touch the head and do not do it for too long, perhaps two or three times a day for a couple of minutes each time. Think of the light green as permeating the baby's whole body, particularly through his lungs, to ameliorate the high degree of irritability and to provide protection from what we might call the mother's vibrations or interactions. Doing TT in this way will help the baby to quiet himself and to stabilize.

Therapeutic Touch for Persistent Pain

When pain persists in spite of apparent healing, it is very difficult to deal with. The physicians will say that there is no residual injury left and there is absolutely no reason for the healed wound to hurt, yet the person remains in pain. From my point of view, the nerves carry the sensation of pain longer than most doctors realize.

TT for Persons with Perceived Pain

TT can help ease perceived pain, a common problem for some people who have chronic pain and who seem to be angry most of the time. First, work with the pain. In this, the projection of healing blue would be very helpful; in fact, saturate the person with it. Then I often work in the healthy area around the problem area, to clear it away. I reinforce areas that are healthy and allow energy to move in to replace or break up the blockages of flow. It is not so much a matter of taking energy away, as it is to get it flowing again. Center deeply, and think consciously of the inner self of the patient. Then, gently but steadily, send out the sense of peace to help the patient reduce his anger and remove whatever is blocking his relationship to his inner self. If you do that in a compassionate, disciplined manner, it can have an effect on the anger within a few days' time.

After a second or third session, the patient may get glimpses of his inner self as he feels better. I do not think it will happen by treating a person once, but it can happen with time. Much of the outcome depends on how long the person has had the pain, as well as any emotional problems that may have arisen.

There are also times when a pain returns even after the nerve supplying that area is cut. The pain may go away, but within a few months it comes back, or it comes back as a slightly different kind of pain. It is baffling because—with the nerves or cord being cut—there is thought to be no way that the pain message could get through. But the body retains the memory of that pain, and the memory feeds back the sensations of pain. Memory has a tremendous influence on the individual, and pain, as memory, has a powerful effect on our ability to survive. By remembering previous painful episodes we are prompted to avoid them. If you are giving a TT treatment, you want to help destroy the memory of the pain as well calming it and treating its effects.

Applying TT to Emotional Distress

If we are sensitive, we unconsciously pick up some of the tensions and the pain of other people and that drains us in many ways. TT therapists also are sensitive to the disturbed feelings of the patients they are working with. It is not easy to pick up another's emotions and keep them in their proper proportion. There are people who are very wild and out of control. When you do TT with them, you may not pick up their feelings in an understandable way, but your own subtle energy fields may quiver, causing you to feel shaken.

From my observations of many accomplished healers, I would say that deep quiet seems to be the baseline requirement for effectiveness. If you are engaged in a healing interaction, caring and compassion are usually called forth automatically. You do not have to consciously turn on those attitudes. However, quietness, calm, and peaceful stability of mind are the result of self-discipline. That is why it is so important that you begin by withdrawing within yourself and making the affirmation, "I *am* that quiet which I feel within." It is a statement of personal belief that each of us has that possibility of quiet and strength within our being. If you have that personal conviction, you can function as a whole even if you are disturbed about something; you can still project the healing energy that arises out of the universal healing energy field. If you can learn to do that even when circumstances are very, very difficult, it will also help in your own stability.

For persons who must go into highly stressful situations daily and want to help others in that situation, I suggest that—before you step into that stressful setting—you stop, center yourself, send out peaceful thoughts, and then open the door. Coming among others in that way, you have a good chance of stabilizing the situation. After you have deeply quieted *yourself,* maintain that discipline and profound quiet while you project a sense of deep peace to the disturbed persons for the period of time it might take to effect a more tranquil atmosphere. You do not have to say anything. You are not forcing anything on them, you are just sending peace to everybody. If there are persons in that group who continue to be disturbed, or are the most disturbed, ask them a question to refocus their attention—it needn't have any sense to it—and continue to send them peace. That unexpected action may open them for a moment so that the projection of peace might enter their consciousness.

You cannot do this if you allow yourself to become disturbed. If someone should shout at you and make nasty remarks, and if you respond heedlessly or angrily, you bring that violence into the healing relationship with the person you are trying to help. It takes discipline not to get upset while in the midst of people who are emotionally agitated. Many times one cannot physically do much for persons who are psychologically disturbed. However, because of the state they are in, they are open, vulnerable, and hypersensitive. They respond to our feelings, most frequently in a manner previously unknown to us. For instance, it may be difficult to recognize why they may suddenly throw a tantrum. Sometimes it is because they have sensed something that they have not understood and they do not feel in control. That is why it is important to calm and compose yourself before you open the door, so that you are prepared. Then the upset people will recognize you as a source of quiet and stability.

If you can maintain that inner state of equipoise as you project a sense of confidence and composure, you can have a remarkable effect on others in a very short time, even under conditions of panic. *But, first the condition must be in you:* the resolute belief or confidence that a center of stillness and unperturbed serenity persists within. That, I think, lies at the center of the ability to help or heal those in need. Although each accomplished healer I have seen was unique and different, all seemed to have that faith in themselves, which they were able to project to others. It does not make any difference whether the healer is conscious of it or not; it can still affect the interaction with the healee.

Although you feel the deepest compassion for the ill person, you will be of more help to them if you go back to the quietness within you for a moment and then send out the healing energy. If you can send them strength out of your own sense of stillness, you can often do a lot to help them compose and quiet themselves without taking all the destructive pain into yourself. If you think clearly of the other person, you can really reach out to him. And that is really the greatest love and the most difficult thing to do.

There is a difference between picking up anger when the healee has lost his temper, and picking up anger that has been mulled over for years. Then the person has made a mental picture. That is a more subtle, but destructive, characteristic because it is partly a mental image as well as an emotional image, and therefore complex. Emotional aspects are in flux, while the image that is made of mental energies is more lasting. But you may be able to affect a patient's mental image by using visualization.

∽◠◉ Using Visualization to Dissipate ◉◠∾
Mental Pictures

Think of mental energies as a light within you, then project that light so that it radiates throughout the person you want to help. This will work also with psychotic people; however, in that case, think of the light more as waves of peace that you are sending them, going from top to bottom of their subtle fields. This is also very helpful if someone is frightfully disturbed emotionally; for instance, if someone has lost a close person by death. Doing TT in this way makes the process more precise.

There is something odd about the reactions of people in the throes of violent emotion: they will automatically reject some of the healing energies. You may have noticed something similar in children when they are intensely disturbed; they do not like something peaceful and reject it. We may unconsciously do the same thing sometimes when we are in a violent temper. If you can calm such patients down, even for a few minutes, they will be better able to respond to the healing.

⟨⟩ Calming a Healee with ⟨⟩
Violent Emotions

However hard it may be to believe until you have experienced it, if you can concentrate and send the healing blue energy to an individual with a fierce temper, you can calm him in just a few minutes. Take a moment, stop the healing, and again think of the light within yourself. Then project it, as royal blue light, toward the healee. This will calm the person from the violence and help him. Such persons are not used to such quieting energies; they are more used to getting violent responses. If somebody sends them peaceful, harmonious energies, it is unexpected, and they respond rapidly. If you send out a positive emotion, such as love, caring, or peace, energy literally goes out of your fields as you send the emotion. This outward flow will protect you from taking in the person's anger as a negative energy.

People who are emotionally disturbed or who have been through a recent trauma are also low in energy. Psychiatric and cancer patients, for instance, need considerable energy and they can drain a more healthy person. In these cases you can use this same practice. In addition, you can remove yourself from that patient's presence by going into another room for five minutes and cutting off connections. It is important for you to physically and psychologically leave that patient. Even if you eventually have to go back, you have the opportunity to restore your normal balance for those few minutes. If you do this consciously, when you go back into the room you will have regained the energy to stop the draining process for some time.

Another aspect of energy exchange can take place when you are working with a patient who—without your being aware of it—becomes very needy for some reason, and reaches you in the solar plexus and drains you.

*ᕦᕤ To Reverse the Feeling of Being ᕦᕤ
Drained of Energy*

*My suggestion would to take a deep breath, which will relax you and
bring oxygen to your brain. For a split second think of energy enter-
ing your solar plexus, and then try to spread it to the periphery of
your vital-energy field. In that way you speed up your own intake of
energy for just a moment; your energy will return to its normal
exchange with the environment and you will feel more in balance.*

Dealing with Anxiety and Fear

If a patient is very confused and anxious, remember that the back of the
neck is the gateway to the brain. That is why we so often suggest that
you go there first when you are assessing a person's problem. You will
usually find two major symptoms. First is the anxiety of the healee
about his illness. In addition, there is the overarching concern of the
mind. The brain is involved also because it makes the connection with
the mind. For example, the patient wonders what the next step of the
disease will be. Such questions are structured through the mind. All of
these concerns act to set up certain patterns—energy patterns, behavioral patterns, and so on—related to how the patient accepts a disease.
These aspects of the patient's struggle with the disease process build up
as muscular and circulatory tensions in the back of the neck, blocking
the flow of vital-energy.

The tension that builds up during pain slows down the effect of
Therapeutic Touch, so you may have to treat the patient two or three
times to work through such a problem. Asking the patient to think of
someone he loves while you are working over the heart center will help
him to break down his attachment to the sickness. The patient's conscious
act of sending love directs the energy flow out of his vital-energy field.

Anxiety sometimes blocks the reception of the healing energies, so
it is important to deal with it early in the TT treatment. If you have
been able to bring some relaxation to the patient, you can ask him to
think of something in Nature, such as a tree, or other object *outside* of

himself. Then, if you send the healing energy to the back of the neck, you may be able to free that person, for the time being, of his anxiety.

Although you have taken away the pain and the healing is accelerating, the healee often slides back into the habit of worrying, even though it may no longer be necessary. To help prevent this from occurring, you can ask the healee, "What worries you the most?" while you are doing Therapeutic Touch. If he answers, suggest that if the same worry recurs, he should immediately recall something cheerful or joyful—something that would bring to mind a picture opposite to that attachment. With chronically ill people, particularly, tell them that such positive thoughts will help them *after a while,* and encourage them in their shifting of energy. If you can help them do this, it will be beneficial, as they, themselves, will see over time.

Treating Persons with Post-Traumatic Stress Disorder

TT can help persons with post-traumatic stress disorder or others with intense, paralyzing fear, but it is not easy and it will not happen in one session. They need to get used to you so that they trust you and can completely relax. After quieting them with TT, you can then ask them what image they would like to think of. Their minds have been caught up in fear and full of negative images, but if they can shift consciousness even for a few minutes, it will help break up that fearful state of mind.

Once trust has been established, you will be able to reach a fearful person by asking him to think of an image that is a reality to him. While you are doing TT, ask him to tell you what most worries him and send him, through your thoughts, a sense of peace. Then have him visualize a symbol that represents spirituality or security to him, and it will bring the sense of peace through. But it cannot be done at once; you must be willing to work with such a person over time.

Some people are so fearful that they cut themselves off from all interaction. To bring this to their attention, I often confront them with the problem. I will say to them, "Of what are you afraid?" If a person is constantly fearful, it is a sign of a disturbed mind. However, if a person gets flashes of fear, it may be an insight or warning about something that is about to happen. The Society of Psychical Research, which has been in existence for over a century, has records of thousands of people who have had such sudden warnings. Often the incident is associated with someone who has passed over. The person who receives the warning is startled and has a sudden fear and stops what he or she is doing and is subsequently saved from an accident or death.

TT *for Emotional Suppression, Depression, and Grief*

Our feelings, and how we use them, are crucial to the development of many modern diseases. The emotions of people who are upset or have strong feelings can become very intense under the pressures of life. As a result, their muscles, particularly in the neck, tighten up as though they were trying to hold back their emotions. Even if it makes them feel upset, they still want to hang on to that disturbed state. They are in a difficult position because they feel so strongly yet they often do not know why and have great difficulty in expressing what they feel. Many of them get headaches or digestive upsets, and the tension can act to bring out a lot of other emotional problems.

Many people whom I meet are chronically tired. They are also depressed because they do not know how to continue their work or other daily responsibilities. In our time it is not unusual for people to feel under pressure ten to twelve hours a day. Therefore, even when they sleep, they do not completely relax, and their worries are always affecting their physical bodies. I feel so sorry for them because their emotional tension brings about so much unnecessary physical pain. It is important to remember that being emotionally disturbed immediately opens a pathway to pain; it is an automatic pathway that reconnects powerfully through the memory. People who are emotionally stressed will either explode or be overwhelmingly drained of energy. Often this is diagnosed as chronic fatigue, but I feel the doctors often do not know what is the matter with the patients, except that they have a low degree of constant vital-energy and they feel tense.

⁄⁄⁄ TT for Depressed Patients ⁄⁄⁄

When a person is very depressed, he turns his energies inward and, to a certain extent, loses his capacity to go out to others and to events. I would suggest that in treating such a person you use a color such as rose and feel goodwill toward him. At the same time, you can think of helping him to open up—that is, release—his energy field, because while it is closed in, the depression will continue. To reach a severely depressed patient who is so inwardly-turned you must focus on opening up the field to free flow. Projecting rose is a good way to try to "break" it open, sensitively and gently. You can also help by visualizing someone you love for a moment, feeling yourself opening to that flow, and sending it to the patient.

Bereavement is not the same as depression, but this technique may be helpful in that case as well. What the bereaved person really needs is for you to care, because in bereavement one feels lonely and even alone in the world. You can help by having a caring attitude and project that feeling toward him in a deep rose.

In the majority of instances grieving lasts for only a limited time. However, there are rare cases where some people hook on to the memory of the relationship. Some years ago a child was brought by her parents to Mr. Estebany. I was startled when I saw that the parents had actually tied their little girl to them by the wrists. It was their pride that made them do that; they were so afraid the child would say silly things. I took her with me and let her wander nearby to her heart's content, and she could say all the silly things she wanted to. She had a wonderful time. Whatever advice was given to the parents had no effect; they would not change their ways. Shortly thereafter the child died. I could not feel sad for the child because in life she had been a prisoner with no opportunity to express herself. The parents went to the girl's grave every day to cry. I do not know if they felt any guilt, but they had deep grief. This is one of those rare cases in which the people may never recover from their loss.

⊸⊘ *Responding to Grief* ⊘⊶

If you are dealing with grieving families or groups and feeling drained, try to listen to something in Nature such as a bird's call or the wind, or visualize a running brook or a tree for a few moments. In that way you will be remembering a sign or symbol of unity, and it will give you a different perspective. Visualizing the symbol will act to lessen the draining of your own energy. Then you can send peace to the family from that frame of mind. Grief can fragment a family, and in this way you can help them to reintegrate as a family unit, while maintaining the integrity of your own field.

Working with People
with AIDS

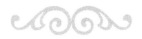

BECAUSE OF CIRCUMSTANCES, I have probably treated more AIDS patients than most healers. I have worked with them in my healing groups and taught them in my classes. They are people in great trouble who are affected by the disease in different ways. One of the symptoms is the feeling that everything suddenly drops out of you, without warning. This overpowering weakness can be very discouraging. Most of them experience so much anxiety and a consequent severe reduction in energy that they are thrown into a depression. The severe depression also brings everything energetic down, truly depressing their functions.

How Therapeutic Touch can help the patient with AIDS largely depends on the patient's state of mind. In general, I laugh a lot when dealing with persons with AIDS. This sounds strange, but it is useful. They are so often tight with anxiety and the laughter gives them the sense of relaxation. The relaxation is a very important ingredient in helping them to achieve a new lifestyle and an acceptance of who they are, in the deeper sense. I recall an amusing story that demonstrates this. One day, while I was treating an AIDS patient, something crossed my mind and I burst out laughing. I think it was the exact thing that needed to be done at that moment. I said to him, "You don't really understand why you are here, and you think this place is a madhouse, don't you?" He laughed and said, "Yes!" and it broke the ice. Before that he had been sitting stiffly and feeling unable to do anything. He felt hopeless; he did not trust his doctors, and he felt they did not know how to treat AIDS. I continued treating him and we talked at length. I then felt that it would be useful to teach him how to do Therapeutic Touch, and he learned how to do TT to others under supervision.

On the last day as I was leaving the hospital I saw him and called out to him, "Hey! You've become part of the madhouse yourself, haven't you!" I had only been there with him for five days, but I could see that a tremendous change had occurred within him. When I first met him he was encased in his own negative feelings, and he was hard to work with because of his refusal to cooperate. I think the process of Therapeutic Touch helped him gain a completely different point of view and a definite psychological shift occurred. As you can see in this story, it is very important to help such patients feel they are making a positive contribution to humanity.

I knew a lawyer who tested positively for AIDS, and the consequences of this testing utterly changed his life. He had earned enough in his law practice that he could help others financially. After being diagnosed, he divided his time between being a lawyer and finding ways to be altruistic on behalf of others. In doing this, he gave up his ambition to be the "best" lawyer. By giving and helping others he discovered what he wanted to do with the rest of his life. Through his acts of compassion he attained a sense of serenity and peace of mind. I admired him very much and thought that he had realized an ideal way of coping with his disease. Working for others made him feel expansive; it made him think of himself as a giving person. In all things he thought not of dying, but of his opportunity to give, which I thought was a very healthy perspective.

Most people come to me when they are first diagnosed, and they are feeling helplessness, anger, and fear. It is a difficult life for the few years before death. I always begin my classes with them by reiterating that it is very important to realize there is a life, an identity, beyond what we experience here and now. I do not say that Therapeutic Touch has saved anyone from death, but when they die, they have changed enormously, from my point of view. Because they have been treated, it has made them peaceful, enabling them to die with a sense of acceptance and often with a quiet serenity.

Many have been part of one of my healing groups for some time where they have been beautifully accepted. We meet regularly, and there is a very close connection within the group. If they are stable, I let them help me to do TT to one of the other patients. Although they may have a very poor prognosis, and it is thought that they will die, being able to give to others transforms these persons immensely. It is very touching to see how being able to give of themselves bolsters their spirit unbelievably. The beautiful part is that they really *can* help, for there are many different ways of giving.

The practice of TT gives them an opportunity for involvement in a spiritual growth process. Achieving the inner quiet necessary to do TT brings the sense of their inner self closer. They come to have a completely different view of themselves. So there is spiritual growth, even for the dying, who are often affected by severe physical pain. Feeling they have done a service to others in need helps them to die very peacefully, without resentment.

Recently one of these friends died. The most accurate word for describing his passing is "beautiful." He had lived his life to the fullest and he accepted his death in peace. Another boy died when he was quite young. He wanted to make a contribution to the world, so just before he died he went to several schools and taught children about AIDS, and his programs were very successful. Everyone gained immense insight through his conscious effort, and he experienced tremendous spiritual growth. He died very peacefully, with his family around him, and amidst the love of many people.

When one of our group of AIDS patients dies, everyone takes time to send that person the message that they care for him or her. For the next three days, they frequently send a sense of caring and love to that person. It makes a difference; it is a service to both the person and to everyone close to them. If a person has a philosophy that accepts death as a natural sequel to life, the effect on the whole group has been astounding. One professor came to us with AIDS. He would not have missed coming to the healing group, because he learned to be at peace, and he eventually died peacefully. Just before he died, he wrote us a letter to say how being in touch with us had meant so much to him. We had a special group commemorative meditation for him. That was his wish.

For many who have been practicing Therapeutic Touch for some time, it comes as a revelation that they have themselves significantly changed during that time. The focus of their lives has shifted, giving them a sense of self-confidence that was not there when they first started practicing. This self-confidence is what is needed to deal with the fear and the sense of crisis about AIDS. Protective gloves are secondary to the kinds of emotions and thoughts you can project to the patient. It is easy to pick up the fear of AIDS that is prevalent in the world and intensified in hospitals today. We get carried away because everyone else is being carried away. Instead, we can say to ourselves, "I am not going to be carried away; I am going to do something to help."

Even if we do this a few times we are making a positive contribution to the atmosphere, instead of allowing ourselves to be swept away by strong opinions that may be verging on panic. We are living in a world where everything seems preordained and it is not always clear that the individual counts, for not much credit has been given to the individual's innate potential for free will. Personally, I feel that the individual does count, and as more individuals act to help others, this contribution spreads. Every individual who works for the benefit of others does more good than he or she realizes.

I have seen Therapeutic Touch practiced under severe circumstances, where we meet regularly. We have doctors helping me, we have nurses helping me, and we have patients helping one another. These meetings with patients who have such great needs help to fulfill a significant function in bringing forth the essence of compassionate healing.

Supporting Persons with Terminal Illness

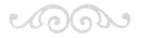

IF YOU ARE IN THE HEALING PROFESSIONS, you are going to have to deal with death, so it is important to learn to accept it. The more you accept it, the more helpful you can be to patients. Healing affects people, not only in keeping them alive but also in the growth of the spiritual self. I think that is an important thing to keep in mind when we deal with death.

There are many reasons for the recent interest in death and the dying experience. Perhaps foremost is that we live in a time and a culture when there are diseases of unknown cause, and a high rate of accidents have come to be accepted as everyday affairs. In addition, there are many more sensitive children born today than we were aware of in former times. Also, of course, death and the dying process have given rise to traditions and events that are the livelihood of many people in our culture. Much research is being done in this area at this time and a great deal of the experimentation has to do with trying to expand or adjust the conventional research to take into account the special conditions in which the dying process occurs.

When a person is dying, he frequently lets go of many of his worries, and his subtle energy fields become less closely knit. Therefore, in a certain sense the person is closer to the inner self, for his fields have been opened. If he becomes well again, that openness gives him the sense of other consciousness or experiences. All patients need to let go, whether they are about to die or not. They are enmeshed in their habit patterns, their attachments and resentments.

I think a person can have a healthy attitude toward his engagement with life in spite of having an incurable disease. I like to conceive of the idea of health as related to wholeness. Wholeness implies being able to function and being organized on all levels of consciousness. A "whole person" not only has physical health, but also emotions that are well integrated and quiet, an excellent, balanced, state of mind, and the capacity to be at peace with oneself.

So many people I know come to mind who—although they may be physically impaired—are nevertheless "whole" because they can see beyond their own immediate needs and give of themselves to others. Some of them have been born impaired, but these people are able to accept it as part of their given life pattern and go on, helping others on the way. They want to help others become aware of the inner self that they have recognized in themselves.

In a real sense, nobody knows when another person is going to die. Doctors may have a considered opinion, but they will admit that nobody knows this with any exactitude. Sometimes the patient has a much firmer idea about his death than do authorities on the subject. Many diseases have their ups and downs, and nobody knows what will happen within the person himself.

I remember an incident that occurred several years ago in Chicago. A young woman who had a very influential position in city government came to see me. She had been diagnosed as having cancer, and she told me that the doctors had given her only two weeks to live. I did not think anyone could be that precise. We talked for two hours, and I gave her some suggestions. She herself was certain that she would continue to work at her present post far beyond the proscribed time. A year later I met the woman's husband who told me that she was alive and even had a promotion in her job. This story underlines that *nobody really knows* when another person will pass on. We are never sure; that foresight is rarely given to us. Let us all take life's changes as they come. Truly, when the time comes, the time comes; you do not have to prepare.

However, many people who are dying are fearful. We can help the dying patient by projecting to them a sense of peace and a sense of flow. By "flow" I mean the acceptance that all of life is filled with constant change. We need to be open to the patients and allow them to talk about death, if they want to. We must learn to allow them to share what they need to share. Even if they have not talked about it, the idea may still be at the back of their minds. Our inner feelings get communicated consciously or unconsciously. If we have a fear, it will be picked up by the patient. But if we can communicate a sense of inner peace and acceptance of the natural flow of all life, we are truly being compassionate individuals.

I remember the first AIDS patient I interviewed. At the time I knew nothing about him. He was considered terminally ill and was naturally full of resentment. We talked for nearly two hours, and while we were talking I was constantly sending him a sense of peace. A year later I was surprised and touched to hear from a friend of his that he felt he had gained a great deal from our talk together. He died peacefully two months after our talk.

We can all help. When a disease is in its very advanced stages and you know there is nothing you can do to heal it, you can still help tremendously by assisting the patient to go peacefully with TT. Remember, everyone has an inner self. Each person experiences this as a deep sense of quietude and peace. We are all linked together in that way. The inner self is very much part of the whole Therapeutic Touch process and it provides an opportunity for the person to grow spiritually. In TT your inner self is contacting the inner self of the dying person. That makes for a beautiful atmosphere in a room. If a person dies in this way, you have done something significant to help him go on.

We must not take it as a personal failure if anybody dies or does not recover from an illness. That is a very difficult thing to learn. As I have said, my personal belief is that certain things in a person's life are predestined. If something is going to happen for an individual and you have given them all you can, you have done your share. In my lifetime I have seen people whose condition has not changed; perhaps they did not want to change. But when they came near death, they suddenly opened up, and they changed. I think TT is helpful in such a circumstance because a TT therapist would be aware of and sensitive to that change. She would know that she could help that person by sending him peaceful and quiet thoughts. Many others would not have the faintest idea about that.

I have seen people really change by being treated with TT for some time. You have to obey doctors' orders, and so on, but with TT you are making your own personal contribution, whether the person dies or not. It is important to accept that dying is not the most terrible thing that can happen. If you can help the person to pass over quietly and with acceptance, both you and that person have made a lot of spiritual progress.

What I am trying to get across is that to help a person die in a state of peace is just as important as being able to help him or her get well. It is not in our hands really, whether a patient stays alive or passes on. Life and death are part of Nature's cycles. If you can offer a patient a sense of peace and be open and quiet, just allowing that person to talk about death, you have achieved something important. If more persons in the health field were able to deal with their own fears about enigmas such as AIDS and death, they would be more truly able to help others. Doing TT makes it easier, because we have a different sense of what is happening.

Many Therapeutic Touch therapists have helped people to die peacefully and to accept it as a transition in consciousness. The word *death* has a fearful connotation in our culture. When we see death as a transition of consciousness, we can help to make that transition peaceful, both for the person who is dying and for their family. The whole family can participate in that transition. I have had letters saying that a family did TT when a relative was sick for a long time; even the children came together to send love and peace to the patient.

The relationship we have to those who have passed on is a personal one and we feel bereft of our communication with them. That is why I suggest to those who are grieving over the death of someone close to them that the love between them will always continue. The one thing the family can always do, instead of crying, is to send that love, and the person on the other side can return that love, too. You can say that to people of any age, and I do not think you would be going against traditions of major belief systems. It gives the family permission to continue to send affection. Then death will not feel like the final end of the relationship. If you can convey this to a grieving family in some way, and a real link is made between the family members, you will have made a valuable contribution to society.

To families whose children have died, I say: "This is the time when they need your love more than anything. If you can send love every day, for a week or two, to that child, you will both be helped, because you can then say to yourself, 'This is forever.' You will know that the relationship continues beyond death."

I tell those who are related to or know any person who has passed on that they should continually send thoughts of caring and of love for three days following the death. It helps the living as well as those who die, because feeling that they are doing something for the person who has passed on eases the time of parting. I am receiving letters from families who have done this saying that it has made a tremendous difference to them to stop saying, "I'll never see them again." Loving a person brings that person nearer. They lose that sense that they have lost them forevermore, and that helps everybody. It is not easy, but it can be done, and it has great meaning for the healer, the family, and the person who has died.

✑ *Dealing with Personal Loss* ✑

Once you are over a loss, it is normal to occasionally feel the pain again when a memory of the person is recalled. Of course you will miss them, but the important thing is to accept the affection that is still there. You can send them expressions of your deep love, and in this way you will never be isolated from each other. Project the color of deep rose if you can, and convey that you care about them and that they are not alone. In that way you are really helping and not being lost in the terrible suffering of your loved one being gone. You are really going out to the inner self of that person, and are giving the enduring love that is between your two inner selves.

Section VI:
QUESTIONS AND ANSWERS

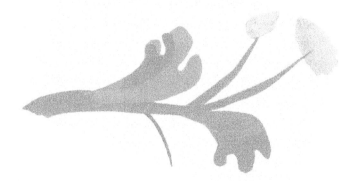

Introductory Comments

Dora was always open to questions; in fact, she encouraged them. She stood ever ready to bridge the enormous gap between the vibrant, constantly shifting multidimensional world of the reality she had known all her life and the dull, dense, tangible 3-D world most of us know. Knowing that our questions would never be considered silly by her gave us tremendous confidence to voice our occasional insights into the frequent psychic phenomena that accompany the healing interaction, itself a largely nonphysical phenomenon.

Another asset Dora possessed that made her an exceptional teacher was the skilled ability to think through complicated or obscure problems, particularly those concerning human relationships, with characteristic directness, lucidity, and candor. For instance, while the idea of the inner self as Dora states it is complex, it is also clear, coherent, and compelling. This is of particular value when teaching a subject such as healing, which deals so intimately with matters of life and death, ultimate issues that are not easy for the novice TT therapist to accept. Over time, as the therapist realizes that she has an ally in the inner self, that recognition generates a surge of confidence that she can handle such serious responsibilities with stability. Very importantly, it also lends her a sense of continuity and an intimation of long-term commitment to helping and healing those in need.

As this sense of the inner self implants itself in a person's activities of living, it touches that life with several indicators of its presence. An increased psychic sensitivity is one early indicator, and this upsurge in sensitivity is often accompanied by synchronous happenings whose timing is awesome. As these abilities are strengthened and become more reliable, the TT therapist often finds herself growing increasingly adept at mind-to-mind communication with the healees with whom she is working. This sophisticated ability—which allows the healer considerable freedom to work in-depth with the healee—takes little physical exertion. It is an effortless effort naturally arising out of her aspiration to help or to heal.

Such increase in sensitivity may take its toll, however, should a therapist mindlessly misuse or overuse her energies—by permitting herself to become overwrought or overfatigued—and thus throw her own self into imbalance. Once this happens, one feels out of the loop, and it takes a very long time to regain that fine-tuned synchronicity with the ten thousand and one events going on simultaneously in one's universe.

On the other hand, if you can maintain your balance—meanwhile undergoing the dynamic personal growth and development that accompanies the inner work of Therapeutic Touch—then life can proceed smoothly, directed by your aspirations. It is as though the universe is behind your efforts, because the results seem greater than the sweat you put into it. To a surprisingly large extent, the body intelligence has its own knowing way of dispersing and dispensing the vital-energy you are making available to the healee during a healing interaction, so that your rate of success is bolstered. Opening yourself to compassionate concern for others in need also is the "open sesame" to the incomparable powers of the heart chakra, thereby significantly increasing the value of your allies in healing. Given your permission to enter into your activities of daily living, the inner self can quicken your finer sensibilities of intuition, aspiration, and insight that mightily fortify your healing ability. Then, when you do Therapeutic Touch with a healee, it "feels right." You work without a sense of effort or fatigue. During the assessment phase you don't know you know until you hear yourself saying the right words at the right time. You choose patients or things to do that nobody else would bother with, and you do it!

What makes this all so easy is that you want to do it, you want to be a healer, you want to help "put together again," to make whole the person you know or the unknown stranger, the event that is nearby or far from you, Humpty Dumpty Who Sits On The Wall or the Cow Who Jumped Over The Moon. You want to help or heal them all because it is right for you to do, now. You, at that in-depth stratum of being known as the inner self, made that decision at sometime in the somewhen and—just as it is the healee's karma to have the opportunity to be healed—it is you, the TT therapist, who has the opportunity to fulfill a karmic decision to help or to heal.

Wanting to heal someone in need puts a person's efforts at a different level of consciousness than merely doing something as a simple response to a modest stimulus, as a social expectation, for example. The aspirational determinant embodies a discerning intentionality, and as such it projects its power from the crown chakra, which can make of the event of healing a truly spiritual experience. However, the stimulus-response reflex springs impulsively from the solar plexus chakra, where one can fall easy prey to overwhelming fatigue and be rapidly drained of energy. In healing in particular, it becomes apparent that each activity, each thought, each behavior has its consequence at an individually appropriate level of consciousness, and one becomes mindful of these nuances.

In our own time we have encountered debilitation to the point of exhaustion in people with AIDS. It is difficult to work with such a person at a physical level because the vital-energy field is so fragile, enervated, and unprotected that it rapidly "leaks" the energy input even as you are working. Dora has worked with more people with AIDS, particularly on the West Coast, than any healer I know. At this writing, however, there are only a few persons with AIDS left from the original TT groups. We never did cure anyone with AIDS, but we could and did help them in the handling of severe crises, especially those concerned with the end stages of final transition. While they were still alive TT significantly helped to reduce or eliminate their pain; we were also able to help them stave off opportunistic infections. However, as Dora notes, the most significant help we gave to them was in teaching them how to do Therapeutic Touch to their peers and allowing them thereby the personal satisfaction of enriching their self-image, which is the optimal reward of this most humane act.

Th̨e Concept of th̨e Inner Self

Question: *Would you briefly restate the concept of the inner self?*

Each of us has a sense of peace and quiet within. Although we are not usually aware of it, I believe that this sense characterizes an aspect of what I call the inner self. Many people call it "soul." I use the term "inner self" because it has no other connotations; it has not been defined.

This inner self has many aspects. One aspect—perhaps the most significant—is a sense of basic unity at the deepest level we can reach. This is the feeling that we are all bound closely together, a sense of genuine brotherhood. In addition to the seeds of peace and quiet within it, the inner self has several levels of consciousness. At the highest level of that consciousness we are all bound together in an orderly process. We all have these different levels of consciousness, which give us access to the many aspects of the inner self.

Each of us is born, lives, and dies, and this is true for all living beings; there is no exception. I personally believe in reincarnation: the inner self comes back life after life. We are here to fulfill certain relationships, and it is in this fulfillment that the inner self learns. The inner self comes into the individual at conception and karma begins to work itself out. From my perspective, even if the fetus dies in utero, that karma has been worked out for the inner self. When a person dies, the inner self continues as a consciousness.

The inner self knows the past history of the individual at its many different levels of consciousness and that its connection with the feeling-thinking personality is at certain times more fully developed, and at other times less so. We are born with certain characteristics that are genetic that have the imprint of the inner self; a few events or circumstances are predestined at birth. How we *act* upon them, however, is not predestined at all. We have the freedom of our individual choice, and that freedom is based in how we accept these various events.

Question: *Can the inner self acknowledge the inner self of another?*

Yes, that is so. If you are well integrated yourself, you can reach people there and help them. During a healing you can acknowledge your inner self and then send the patient energy at that more subtle level. There is this recognition: *Here is someone who knows that I am that inner self and who understands what I am going through.* A dying person particularly needs that sense of companionship when the end of life is approaching. There is no use in talking of it in an intellectual way to a person who is very sick. It is a difficult concept to grasp, even under ordinary conditions. Even while a person's inner self is responding to you, the concept is not within the popular cultural frame, in the more rational sphere, and they may have a difficult time perceiving it. Still, this type of mind-to-mind, silent communication is as much care as anyone could give. We should think about it and consciously use it more often in our care giving. It may be the most subtle and difficult thing to do, but the ability can be cultivated.

Most of the experiences that we have of direct communication with the inner self while we are healing are "smaller" experiences than the engagement one has when there is a profound sense of the unitary nature of the universe. The latter can be a deep mystical experience. The encounter we may have while healing someone who is ill is more like having a glimpse or seeing a reflection of the inner self. The mystical experience is more rare, whereas identifying with a level or aspect of the inner self is more common, and this is what we do well during Therapeutic Touch.

Therapeutic Touch

Question: *Many people are curious to know what is happening energetically when we are working on a patient. When we are doing Therapeutic Touch, it seems like something is happening, but to describe it, I think we would be hard put.*

What we are trying to do in Therapeutic Touch, first of all, is to give the person enough energy at the level of the physical body to strengthen the immune system. In this way the body itself can fight the disease and self-healing can take place. When I look at a person, I see the physical body as well as the rhythms of the different energy flows of all the physical organs. Interpenetrating that is the person's *life-energy*, the energy that keeps the whole body going in a rhythmic function. Interpenetrating that are feelings. You *know* feelings are energy, don't you? Just think of when you get angry! When we experience our own emotions, which we are feeling all the time, we are also building patterns. If we repeat something a thousand times, the energy is built up in those feelings each time we repeat it, and these energy flows are directive.

So, each person has different levels of consciousness. First there is the energy in regard to the physical body, then the energy of the emotions. Then there is the energy present in that level of consciousness where people *purely* think. Then comes what I call the intuition, the level where one connects more with one's inner self. This is operating when a person suddenly gets flashes of inspiration or intuition. We experience the last level of consciousness at times in meditation, when we feel a sense of complete unity with other human beings and Nature. I call this the deepest level of the inner self. All of these levels act upon us *all* the time and make up our personality.

In the healing you are sending energy; you project a healing energy *through* you. I think first of the energy of your physical body, and also of emotions. During the Therapeutic Touch the healing energy coming through you sends strength through the physical area in the patient where there is disease. If you know of the disease, and you think of that area of the physical body as being balanced, this helps the healing. But the patient's body will pick that energy up and put it where it's most useful even if you do not know what the specific disease process is.

If you practice Therapeutic Touch regularly, that will help bring all the different levels of consciousness into harmony, fostering heightened perception, more flashes of intuition, a greater sense of unity—all these things that are part of your own consciousness, because you are linked up to the energy of the universal healing field. You call upon it when you think and project and do the healing. You draw that universal healing field down through you, and you are the channel. You can call it whatever you like, but you can call upon it. In fact, all of us call upon that field, everyone in every country, of whatever religion. That is why you need to be quiet and peaceful for a moment before you begin Therapeutic Touch.

Question: *Why is centering so important in Therapeutic Touch?*

What most people automatically do when they want to help another person is to open up and take the other within themselves. This is a natural thing and one of the reasons for nurses' burnout. If you open yourself in that way, the people you are working with will all be needing energy, and your energy will be drained. Centering is learning to do the opposite.

First of all, it begins with a pattern you establish within yourself. You think of your energies focused in your heart for a moment or two until you feel very still. When you have within yourself the sense of quietness—which very often really is the metaphor for wholeness—then you deliberately send out a sense of caring and wanting to heal other people. Then the patients cannot drain you so much because you are focusing your consciousness at a different level from where they drain the energy. It is a protection for yourself that is also helpful to the patients.

Once you center within yourself, it is easier for you to be an instrument for healing while projecting this sense of wholeness. That will enable you to be compassionate to the pain and distress the other person is feeling, while realizing that patients' views are often distorted. Recognizing that you can be an instrument of healing energy also has a positive effect upon you, giving you a sense of confidence in yourself that few people have.

The first part of centering has nothing to do with being a channel but is something you do completely for yourself. If you do it often enough, it becomes automatic. You gather your energies, your focus of consciousness, and just *be still*. Get yourself in focus. When you have felt this moment of quietness within, then only—again, for one moment—think of yourself as being an instrument.

Question: *Why does TT work so quickly to produce a relaxation response?*

It seems that there is a lot of tension at the base of the brain and you can easily access that area. That is why we recommend beginning at the back of the neck. Although the front or anterior part of the human body has many structures that lend themselves to relaxation or have a calming effect, such as the carotid arteries, the heart, the solar plexus, the gastrointestinal tract, and so on, TT done on the front does not get as rapid a response. Doing TT on the area at the back of the neck evokes an immediate relaxation response throughout the entire body, and that is the way to visualize it as well, as a whole-body response. Several clinical studies have confirmed that a relaxation response can reliably occur within four minutes when the Therapeutic Touch process is used. It may not necessarily affect pain, if the person has it, but the healing itself will occur much faster if the body is relaxed.

Question: *Can we do TT effectively on our own family members?*

It takes self-discipline to work with one's family members. As much as you want to help, you will not be such a good healer because of the closeness of your relationship with the patient. However, you can try. You should acknowledge that you are attached to the outcome and actually say to yourself: "I am attached." It is normal to be attached, but before doing TT, give yourself two or three minutes to be very calm and show your love by doing TT in a disciplined fashion, and then try to help to the extent that you are able.

Question: *In your opinion, what part does compassion play in the ability to be a healer?*

That is a difficult question to answer because, finally, what is compassion? To take Mr. Estebany—a well-known healer with whom I worked—as an example: his first effort at healing happened because he really loved the horse assigned to him while he was in the cavalry of the Polish Army. The horse had fallen and broken his leg. According to Army rules, he was to be killed in the morning. Mr. Estebany stayed in the stable with the horse all night, rubbing his leg, gently stroking him, and praying for him. In the morning the horse's leg had healed, and he lived for many years. I suppose that the horse and he had achieved a certain unity.

I have talked with a lot of famous healers; however, of them all, Mr. Estebany developed his healing ability in the most unique manner. There was no religious motivation, for instance; there was just a genuine outflow of compassion. This compassion released within him an overflow of affection, which we look upon as a human energy. In stroking that horse's leg all night long, he gave direction to that energy and to the energy bound up in his earnest wishes for the horse to be well again.

Mr. Estebany was a very simple-minded, straightforward man and he carried this simplicity into his healing, particularly when he worked with children. It was very apparent that in the background of his mind he wished the children to be whole, to be unimpaired, in a general sense. He had an exceptional flow of energy and, when he thought about the ill or hurt person, he unconsciously drew on that universal healing energy, which responded instantaneously to the depth of his compassionate thoughts.

Therefore, I would say that compassion plays a number of roles during healing. It helps to bond and unify the healer and the healee. It also has a channeling role: the force of compassionate concern coming from the therapist's heart chakra draws directly from the universal healing field and targets the healee for the flow of healing energies. A very important part of that healing moment is the image that the healer holds of the healee as being whole and unharmed.

Question: *Do the auras of people with the same disease show the same patterns in them?*

No two people are the same. The disease patterns of their physical bodies may be similar, but they are not identical. And the emotions and other fields are very different. The patterns depend on the stage of the disease, the amount of damage to the organs, how long the person has been fearful, and a dozen other considerations.

Question: *Would the pattern of a future illness be seen in a child's aura?*

I do not think so. I think I could pick up a child's destiny, her abilities, and her basic nature, but I do not think I would know the details. When I did a series of studies on the medical inferences of patterns in people's auras, I never saw some of those people again, so I have no further data on them. Of the few babies I saw, I felt at the time that I could perceive only part of their future; in my book, *The Personal Aura* (1991), I update and document that material.

Specific Conditions

Question: *Does TT lend energy to cancer?*

I think it is nonsense to think that doing TT to a person with cancer could give energy to the cancer. When we do TT, our intentionality, our mind, is constantly focused on letting the cancer go and healing the body so that it is strong enough to reject the disease.

Question: *In your opinion, are there specific organs we should work on in the case of malignancy?*

As always, the back of the neck should be worked on. When doing Therapeutic Touch with patients with any malignancies, I would emphasize that you work on the site of the liver, as well as working on the front of the healee. The dysfunctions are basic in many disease processes, and particularly in the malignant diseases. In addition, the liver has a great deal to do with numerous body functions such as the immune system.

The lungs, of course, are very basic and should be worked on, whether from the front or the back. Lung function is concerned with our breathing, and our primary access to prana. If the healee complains of extreme frequent or chronic fatigue, that is a sign of a blockage to lung function. Working on the solar plexus as well as the lungs in these cases will be most helpful, because of the extreme stress and prolonged periods of pain often experienced by persons who have malignancies.

Question: *Why can't Alzheimer's disease be healed by the inner self?*

In persons with severe Alzheimer's the inner self is not really closely associated with the personality, so that the whole consciousness is not aware of pain, for instance. Therefore, if they are asked to do something, only a half or part of the total person responds. With Alzheimer's, the person increasingly loses the sense of "I am directing it" in relation to activities, particularly the "I am" part. Whatever they feel for the moment, they act out.

How can we help? If it is your father or mother, I suggest that three times a day you put your hand on the back of the person's head for one minute, while you are feeling and projecting a sense of order and peacefulness to him or her. It will have an effect, but it will not last long. I don't suggest this for hospital patients, because you would have to do TT to them more often than you would have time for in a hospital.

Question: *I work with a lot of elderly people and many of them are diagnosed with Alzheimer's. They may have unresolved issues. What would you recommend to do with TT?*

I would like to work with some people who are newly diagnosed with Alzheimer's, for the problem in their energy fields would be clearer. Of course, there is a slowing down in the brain. I am not an expert, but I would put my hand over the heart chakra and particularly work on the top of the head and ask the patient to visualize a common thing—the very simplest thing. If he can do that, then his mind is functioning in an integrated fashion.

Question: *I work with some Alzheimer's patients when they are agitated. As soon as I stop TT, they become agitated again. What causes this?*

It is because you are not reaching the lower, deeper part of the brain but only reaching their basic feelings. The mind has to be able to function as a whole. If you could help them in the way I just described, it might help to delay the full effects of Alzheimer's.

Question: *What are your suggestions for doing TT with a person with a diagnosis of Parkinson's?*

Something like what I suggested for the Alzheimer's patient would work, but I would work farther down the body too. Because of the tremor, it is important to direct energy through the arms and the hands. The brain is connected with the tremor in the hands. If the tremor is very slight, the disease is working itself out in a minor way. If the tremor is slight, it is less important than damage elsewhere; in that case, I would work elsewhere and leave the tremor alone. Do not make quick movements if the disease is advanced. If the patient has had Parkinson's for some time, I would be *very* slow.

Question: *And if the patient is being treated with drugs for Parkinson's?*

I would still do the same and see what happens. When I first treated the patient with Parkinson's whom we are working with this week, he had absolutely no sensation in his legs. The next day he had sensation. He could feel heat and cold. He could feel the ground. In other words, his sense of touch had come back. So we have done something for him. Although I have only treated him twice, he is a different person, beginning to feel himself in control. This is primarily because I am making him sit up straight and breathe consciously. It has made an enormous difference to him, because he does not breathe properly. Getting plenty of oxygen is a very important thing. I am very pleased with his progress.

Question: *How would you work with people with psychological problems?*

That is difficult. Such patients are very sensitive to other people's emotions. However disturbed the patient is, you have to be very calm; you cannot be agitated in any way. That is the most important thing, for otherwise you do not help them at all. You can calm down people who are very set in emotional disturbances, but you must keep in mind that the nature of the disease may result in their having distorted impressions. Do TT several times over a period of time. It takes a longer time because the distortion becomes part of their automatic emotional response, and that really affects their basic perceptions. I have talked to people who are doing TT more frequently, who say the patients like it after a while. The distorted ideas may come, but they respond after three or four times.

Question: *Can TT be used with psychiatric patients at a distance?*

Such patients are very much harder to handle than a patient who is in physical pain. You can take away pain in a few minutes. Psychological problems take more time because the nerves and circuits are set in distorted patterns. If you get a distorted reaction, do not be disappointed. That is natural. Some people meditate before they are going to treat a psychiatric patient and then project healing energy to them. You can talk calmly to them while you think of peace and tranquility within yourself. With every word, send tremendous healing energy toward them. It is a slow process. Maybe in time they will allow you to touch them from the back. If you do something from the back, the intervention then becomes impersonal. It is very important for you to be absolutely quiet and clearly send them waves of quietness. I have been in touch with nurses who have tried this in very small institutions. They say that it takes time, but it quiets the patients down, and the patients like it. If they can accept that, you have made the first step.

Question: *Is there anything that can be done at the energy level for persons with AIDS?*

I think we can help them a great deal with Therapeutic Touch. We have experimented with many ways of doing that. Within bounds, we can help them physically, and we certainly have helped them emotionally. I personally have worked with more than seventy-five persons with AIDS at this time, and I will continue to do so. My experience has not been immense, but it has been concentrated.

We have had many people with AIDS come to our annual invitational Therapeutic Touch workshops for health professionals so that nurses and doctors can learn how to deal with these problems. Then the professionals go back to their hospitals and work with their patients with AIDS, often developing a Therapeutic Touch team just for that purpose. In addition, the persons with AIDS also learn to help themselves, and the results never fail to amaze me. In general, they are doing well, they are working, and they have a positive attitude toward their experiences.

For some, the intervals between crises lengthen after a long time of intensive work. As an example, let me tell you of one person who has had positive results. He has been coming to our workshops for four years, and he says that his doctors have taken him off all medication and he has no symptoms. He is an exception; most of the others have not had such dramatic revisions in their condition.

I think people with AIDS could help both themselves and others in a similar predicament by holding conferences on ways in which they could help each other. I can see in my workshops that they do help one another when they come together and do Therapeutic Touch to each other. It is a tremendous boost to them physically and emotionally. When I first started to work with all these persons with AIDS, they did not think they were contributing much by coming together into groups. I was very touched by what one of them later said to me. He said that never in his life had he experienced such peace, such ability to help another person, and such a renewal of self-confidence.

Our workshops are operated as a large community, and everybody pitches in to help the camps operate. The mix of staff, health professionals, and patients is a healthy one, and the experience adds to their sense of self-confidence in being a functioning member of a societal unit again. It is this sense of being a contributing member of society that is so healing. They leave with a sense of self-confidence that they may not ever have had before, and they are better able to deal with later periods when they feel depressed. It is the isolation that they feel, their sense of uselessness, that is so disheartening to them. Each person can do something, not spectacular perhaps, but something that is helpful to someone else, to the community.

There are very few people in the world who really want to help others. If you are dedicated to really helping people in need and to centering your consciousness on the sense of peace and stillness of the inner self whenever you have the chance, you can make a difference, even for persons with AIDS. It takes discipline as well as compassion, but you will see a tremendous difference in your life. If I think of the thousands of nurses who have gone through our workshops, and the decidedly different human beings they now are, I see that they have learned the act of giving to others. They have a sense of dedication to that giving, the self-confidence that they can really help others, and the realization that to be the best caregiver, you first of all have to achieve peace of mind within yourself.

Question: *What is the most helpful way to work with someone who is actually in the dying stage?*

You don't *give* them energy, that's the first thing. You just think of them being peaceful, all over, and of *very slowly* letting them go with peace. I personally have this absolute feeling that the dying process is a very natural process. If the people around the dying person send love and let that person go, it makes the process easier. If a person is very, very ill, let him go. You may miss him in the physical world—there's no doubt about it; but he has been greatly helped by you in his dying process if he can relax.

By accepting the idea of the inner self and that the inner self of the other person has accepted the outcome, you can then reach out to him from that place of acceptance. Think of your inner self, reaching out to the inner self of the dying person, and silently send the thought, "Peace will come." If you send either blue or peace—not *giving* them energy—simply enveloping them in blue, for instance, this can be helpful. I think you can reduce the pain.

Just let Nature take its course. Nature has established a way long ago, isn't that so? If there is a physical obstruction, then send healing energy through that area. The person is dying, so the inner self is leaving; so just be peaceful and allow that to happen. The more calm you are, the more peace *you have,* the more you can be of help to the dying during their final transition.

In America, more than in some other countries, I think there is a horror of death; in hospitals, death is the ultimate enemy. But death actually is a normal process. There is no living thing that does not die. This is a law of the universe. I personally believe that the inner self survives death. I don't say it is the truth; it is what I believe.

As TT therapists, we can contribute during the dying process. If you help people to achieve peace of mind, you are really helping their spiritual growth, to some extent. Therapeutic Touch has helped people to die peacefully, because they have been sent thoughts of peace and letting go. This is very different from the terrible anxiety, projected in some instances by family members, which tries to keep them alive till the last minute. I think that to allow someone to die is very unselfish and a real test of love.

Question: *You often make the statement, "The outcome is not in our hands." Could you speak about that?*

The outcome of nothing is in our hands. We do not decide when or how a person dies; we are not masters of anybody's destiny. We can be helpful and do our best, but more we cannot do.

You cannot be a good healer until you learn this. You have been given an opportunity to help, and you may have a tremendous effect, but you're not the driver—remember that. Then you will not get tired out, feeling sad that you haven't succeeded. You accept your limitations, and that is an important acknowledgement.

You have to give all the caring and help that you can, but you cannot eliminate something from somebody else; they have to be willing to cooperate with that. And if they don't, it is not in your hands. You have to accept that you may never know the scope or the degree to which somebody else will accept your help. That is their decision. This is a very important lesson to learn. Otherwise, you have a misconception of the universe, thinking that it is in your hands. *It is not in your hands.*

Negative and Positive Energy

Question: *Can we work with our own vital-energies to change patterns of negative emotions, such as irritation or anger?*

I think that awareness is the way to stop them, isn't it? Very often we are not at all aware of how often we repeat a negative pattern. But the moment you have that awareness, I think you have begun. Once you have made up your mind to change, you can do it, because it is uncomfortable to feel anger, isn't it?

If you have a pattern of feeling angry, you need to ask yourself, "Why am I so angry?" I recommend actually keeping a notebook for two weeks, writing down how angry you are, and how often. That will give you an insight into your own violent feelings and the cause of them. Then, when you notice that you are feeling angry, try to sit absolutely still and say, "I know I'm angry now, but"—and you must say this—"I don't wish to be." That is the beginning of changing the pattern. After being quiet, reach out to that person energetically, and within yourself silently say "I'm sorry for that." With these words, send out a sense, a thought, of peace to the person.

Sometimes you both love and hate the person you have injured. Try to say to yourself, "I am quiet now. I let my anger go. Let me just make up for that thought of hate by centering and feeling a sense of quietness." A person who has been hurt by your violence needs a moment to feel your changed thought. So you don't need to say anything. A period of quiet—just sending a sense of calmness and not talking—can build a relationship. Sometimes there is really nothing to say, isn't that so?

Sometimes you know that you should change, but you don't want to. It does not sound logical, but even if you want to change, you can be caught in a habit pattern of doing things a certain way. Intellectually, you may realize the need for change, but you have gotten comfortable with the things you do, even though they make you feel uneasy. All of us do this to some extent. It is human to like uncomfortable patterns of behavior, for sometimes they make us feel alive; that is one way of putting it. The question is, how *are* we going to change?

If you take it too seriously, you may set up a condition of conflict. I suggest that you say to yourself, "Here I am, at it again!" and laugh at it. If you can laugh at it, slowly you will not mind changing. Even being able to laugh at it lessens the attachment that you have to that pattern. If you make it a deep conflict, then you will have an internal confrontation, and you will probably rationalize yourself out of making the change.

I think meditation can be very helpful in breaking a pattern and in starting a new one, a positive one. If you become aware when you have been sharp to another person and upset him, you can consciously stop it by sending the calming blue energy we use in Therapeutic Touch toward that person. Doing that in a meditative, quiet way, can alter the disturbed emotions between people.

Question: *I am not given to introspection. How can I become aware of my negative emotions?*

First of all, center yourself. Then, bring to mind a person who most disturbs you. Realize that you have a disturbed memory of that person and accept that. Then, withdrawing your energies and centering them in your heart, think of that person again. Send him a calm feeling as blue light. Then be still for one minute and see if the disturbing image can be quieted down. Think of that memory or of the image of that person as going out. You can envision it as moving out of your thoughts and feelings while you feel the sense of peace of your center and say to yourself, "*I am that peace,*" or "*I am that self,*" so that you get a sense of focus.

Question: *Can resentment make a person feel physically ill?*

The stress of resentment can affect the immune system. A good many illnesses are made worse, or recovery is slowed by resentment. It is not the originator of all disease, but it can prolong a chronic illness. Also, if there is a genetic weakness in an organ, resentment could affect that organ first, since it is low in energy.

Question: *How can we personally deal with resentment?*

Resentment is often generated by setbacks one has in the early years. The emotions become so deeply seated and habitual that we are unaware of the extent of our resentments. Automatically, without thinking, we come back to a picture of pain and resentment, and immediately we are caught up in that pattern. We do not realize that now we are very different individuals and that pattern does not have to mean so much to us anymore. Instead we should say to ourselves: "All right, there is that pattern, but here I am and I am very different."

Most of us have developed a lot of strength within. Events have shaken us like a tree in a very strong wind, but we are much more rooted than we think. So take yourself in hand and acknowledge: *"This was a part of my life.* However, I, at this moment, can say, *it has nothing to do with me as I am now."* If it has to do with a person, visualize that person being some distance from you, and send that person goodwill. The realization that *you* are such a different person is the first important thing.

People often feel resentment if they do not get sympathy for whatever emotional reactions or ideas they have. When we listen to other persons' difficulties, they often may not seem so very important. It is then hard to feel sympathy and the person reciting his difficulties may be deeply hurt. There is so much uncertainty in this world today, and it is common that people who are feeling uncertain want to unburden themselves of their doubts. We as listeners can simply say, "I understand there are many people who share uncertainty in the country right now, and they share your concern," and send out thoughts of quietude and peace to that person. That will help them to compose themselves and perhaps to look at their problems from a fresh perspective, letting go of their resentment.

Question: *Can you say something about the special energy of music?*

Music has energy at a different level than that with which we usually interact, and some people are tremendously affected by it. The sound of music sends energy and the reflection of this energy deeply within has profound meaning to them. When I lived in New York I became very closely connected with some well-known musicians. After the son of a world-famous pianist had committed suicide, the father asked me to come to a gathering of musicians. Some were quite old, others were quite young, but music meant everything to them. I felt very much out of place because I was the only outsider among all the accomplished musicians. However, he had asked me to come, and I couldn't refuse. What I found very interesting was that, although they all were very upset by the boy's death, they talked about nothing but music. That is how they consoled themselves and kept their grief under control. It was language that spoke to them deeply from within.

It was a very new experience and a very valuable lesson for me to realize this unusual level of communication. I realized that we, as a culture, underestimate such people and also people in the arts. Life gave me this opportunity to meet people who were absolutely possessed by the sound of music, and it gave me an insight that I don't think I would ever had otherwise. In my book on the human aura (*The Personal Aura,* 1991) I describe some of the musicians I knew. Nothing else mattered to them. Maybe some people feel that way about baseball, but I don't really understand baseball, so I am speaking from a prejudiced point of view. However, I can see that such an intense interest—whether in music or baseball—lifts people beyond themselves and opens their mind along a special track of thought. For a person who is open to it, it is really an experience in consciousness, whether we speak of audiences in a concert hall or crowds in a ballpark.

THE ANGELIC
KINGDOM AND
HUMANITY

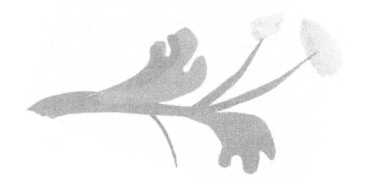

Introductory Comments

Shortly after one of Dora's books, *The Real World of Fairies* (Kunz, 1977), was published, I congratulated her on its success. An odd far-off look came to her eyes and she quietly said, "It's strange that people more quickly believe in fairies than they believe in angels." Something in her tone of voice was so poignant that I found myself avoiding her gaze. Recalling that incident, I realize that attitude toward the reality of angels is still prevalent even these many years later, although all the major religions in the world include a concept of angels in their belief systems and mention legends about them in their traditional holy writings or creation stories.

Perhaps some of these disclaimers are a product of our pragmatic age, in which "seeing is believing" and not many of us are actually able to see nonphysical objects or beings. I am one such person. However, something can translate itself when we are in the presence of such intelligences: we "get a feeling" that is experienced in a singularly palpable manner. Although the experience seems confusing and we may have difficulty describing what occurred, it is most frequently an unforgettable experience, and it often imprints itself on our attitudes thereafter. My conviction that such can be the case rests on several personal experiences, one of which concerns Dora.

One summer day Dora and several of her students, I among them, went to an area of the Berkshire Mountains in Massachusetts, which had over one thousand acres of high blueberry bushes. There was an abundant crop that year and we picked (and ate!) the ripe, juicy berries for several hours. Finally it was time to get back to camp and Dora—with her unusual gait that could cover large tracts of ground exceedingly quickly, her feet seemingly never actually touching the earth—assumed the lead. Happily for me, I could then walk rapidly too, so I was privileged to fast-walk with Dora, loaded berry pail hanging from each hand.

In a very few moments we were perhaps a hundred yards ahead of the rest of the group as we came down the mountain at a fast clip. We topped a knoll, on the other side of which was an extensive white birch grove. To my utter surprise, as I looked at the birch trees, the sunlight seemed to be transposing into a subdued, somewhat misty, yellow-green light, which, nevertheless, was vibrant with a sense of rejoicing and liveliness. I found myself suddenly coming to a standstill, transfixed by I knew not what. Dora's stride carried her a few yards ahead, but she stopped and said, "What is the matter?" to which I could only reply, "Oh! it is so beautiful!" Dora looked at me as though I was a bit daft, glanced in the direction of my gaze, at the sun-dazzled birch trees, and simply said, "Yes, it is beautiful," and continued her stride, me hurrying after her.

Dora never said another word to me about this incident; however, some years later I was listening to one of her tapes, which had been recorded on the West Coast several weeks after the occurrence noted above. She had been giving a workshop on angelic life, and in the recorded talk she described in detail the many interesting activities in which the angelic and fairy life of that birch grove were engaged when we came upon them. I was stunned by the information. For me, it had been only a fleeting moment of idyllic charm: the birch trees were only birch trees, the curiously diffuse luminosity of the sunlight could be explained by Physics 101 and the small, inarticulate voice deep inside could be easily ignored in the incessant rush to do the next scheduled thing.

I had looked at that remarkable tableau, but I did not "see" it. However, several such happenings subsequently served to firm up my decision to accept the existence of angels as an assumption, for their reality certainly had as much validation as other clinical studies in which I had been engaged. For instance, over the years I came across a rich transcultural literature that went back to most ancient times. A more modern, highly credible evidence of record was also being gathered—including repeated sensory data regarding feelings, impressions, and experiential information on intimations of angelic presence—that could form a plausible base for future investigation. This frame of reference freed me, for instance, to accept that my first friends when I was a child were trees and that I continue to maintain those relationships. I have written about these interactions elsewhere (Krieger, 2002) for this assumption has become very much part of my own healing way, though—as Dora correctly remarks in this section—belief in angelic presence is not a part of the teachings of Therapeutic Touch.

However, it is easy to be impressed that there is reality behind the notion of angelic presence when one has had a great deal of experience with healing or being in environments that attract angelic presence, such as hospitals, particularly their crisis centers, such as trauma rooms or labor and delivery rooms, or in hospices. This sense of angelic presence is particularly striking around the major religious holidays, so much so that when I was working as a clinical nurse I preferred to work during the Christmas and Easter holidays, for it was then that exceptional circumstances regarding critical situations were available, more so than at other times of the year. One could witness for oneself the testing of this assumption of angelic presence time and again, not only in cases of unexpected and extraordinary or unprecedented life-saving interventions, but also in the sudden change in the affect of patients who were in the throes of final, often painful, transition. A sense of calmness, composure, and peacefulness would descend upon the dying person like a welcome deep sigh of relief. Just a moment of profound quiet, and then the person's consciousness was decidedly altered, changed irreversibly in that quiescent silence, and only a feeling of gratified fulfillment or tranquil serenity diffused through the room to mark the pervading sense of angelic presence that seemed to assist and accompany their passing.

Relationships between angels and human beings occur most naturally at that profound level of consciousness that is in touch with the inner self. The essential conditions for making contact with them are few: have an overriding interest in helping others, be emotionally stable, reflect a sense of internal mindfulness in outward actions, and demonstrate a willingness to exert self-discipline. Nonetheless, "the trouble about communicating with angels is us" says Dora unequivocally, for we most often focus exclusively on our own thoughts, perseverate our habit patterns, and then lose the opportunity for intuitive hints from the inner self. During TT these intelligences can come to the therapist's aid if several conditions are met: the communication itself must be clear, compassionate concern for the healee's well-being must be strong, the intentionality of the healing act needs to be explicit, the healee's karma must allow it, and the need must be urgent for nonordinary intervention. When they do help, they do so in a manner that is appropriate to the individual person and we can sense their help in our uplifted feelings. However, Dora advises, the TT therapist should first try her utmost to help or to heal the ailing person, and to think of the angels as supportive background for what she, herself, can do.

In accepting the assumption of angelic presence, one also has to accept the responsibility to resist engaging in fantasy. It is not that engaging in fantasy is either a right or a wrong thing to do. However, when a healer is engaged in healing, she is intervening in someone else's life and is therefore committed to maintaining an object-oriented reality base for what she claims to be doing. Under these circumstances, the criterion is the prevalent consensus reality and the healer must be willing to be guided by the social mores of her time.

Our time is, admittedly, a difficult one, partly because our culture has taken so long to see beyond a value system heavily weighted towards materialism. Consequently, "feelings," which are the basis for a belief in angelic presence for most of us, are not considered to represent reality unless they can be measured or coded according to some generally accepted standard. Avoiding the tired question, "How many angels can stand on the head of a pin?" and cutting to the chase, the decisive point regarding the concern about the "reality" of angelic presence is that an argument based on present-day, still heavily object-oriented standards is nonsensical, since the context in which our current, barely extended, three-dimensional standard of reality has been developed does not conform to that other-dimensional realm in which angelic presence could claim validity.

Thus, we have a double-edged dilemma. For many people that parallel state of being remains unreal. For those of us who feel we have had an experience of angelic presence, how do we answer perhaps the most poignant question humans have asked themselves through the ages: "How do I know?" Once we've felt and noted the uniquely stunning effects of angelic presence, how do we get beyond the transverbal, "Wow!"

The experiential knowledge that flows from the Therapeutic Touch healing interaction leads to a personal knowing. As Dora notes, as we affirm the presence of the inner self in our lives, concomitantly we gain insights that illuminate the TT process. In the course of integrating the inner self, there is an increased appreciation of subtle energies and their dynamics and one becomes awake to the multiple realities that surround their world. As the TT therapist grows in experience and purposefully decides to begin this journey by permitting her inner life to fuse with and charge her outer life or persona, Therapeutic Touch becomes for her a transpersonal act. It is then that the therapist accepts transpersonal interactions such as angelic presence as a valid assumption. Admittedly, this is based on personal knowledge, but she works with it, keeping one eye ever alert for effects on the healee that might credibly reflect angelic presence, and the other eye always cautious for his safety and well-being.

Jean Houston, the noted author, states the dilemma well (*Life Force*, 1993) when she says that "today is a time between parentheses," a time caught between changing paradigms or models. For the past quarter century, at every turn worldwide—politically, economically, socially, educationally, industrially, militarily—there has been a contest for radical change between factions of rigid, self-limiting, mechanistic, and reductionist thinking and proponents of a new vision of reality that gives emphasis to a vista of vital interconnectedness and relationship, dynamic patternings, and continual, revitalizing change and transformation. There is a mutual unease about this confrontation; nevertheless, the time is upon us when there is a felt urgency to open ourselves to new and different insights.

Carl Jung, the eminent psychoanalyst of the twentieth century, called the past decade an End Point, for it was not only an end of a century, but of a millennium. It is time, Jung said, for a radical shift in perception; it is important, even crucial, that we think in new ways. Christopher Fry, a foremost poet of our time, says it a bit differently, perhaps with a note of exasperation: "Will you wake, for pity's sake," he exclaims (*A Sleep of Prisoners*, 1951). "Now is the time to wake up . . . We must act as if what we do makes a difference."

One of the seminal ideas that has come out of this plea for a fundamental shift in the perception of our reality has been the introduction of high level functioning where the natural potentials of being are quickened and actualized. This level of consciousness is called transpersonal because it allows one a perspective that is beyond the usual view of reality: a nonordinary perception. This is the level of consciousness the mature TT therapist strives toward, and it is within this transpersonal context that an assumption of angelic presence is cogent and is credible.

Several of the recognized leaders in the development of the concept of the transpersonal would support these assertions. Briefly, Stan Grof's extensive studies on transpersonal states of consciousness (Grof, 1988) demonstrate that these experiences seem to ". . . tap directly into sources of information that are clearly outside the conventionally defined range of the individual . . . and span an immense uninterrupted experiential continuum." Ken Wilber (Wilber, 1980), in laying the groundwork of transpersonal experience, clearly speaks to the difference between transpersonal experiences and perceptions that are in fact pre-personal and often immature; for example, instinctual, infantile, impulsive, and self-assertive, which are traits more typical of regression to narcissistic absorption. However, he says, transpersonal, transegoic states are characterized by increasing self-realization and a more elevated, spiritual state. Finally, in this brief overview, in summation of his years of seminal studies on transpersonal states of consciousness, Charles Tart (Tart, 1981) concludes that transpersonal experiences are potential in human beings and arise from the deep unconscious. His studies strongly imply "that human consciousness may not always be restricted to the body or the brain," and he makes the case that "there may be other kinds of consciousness than human with which we can interact."

All of the foregoing statements were made by persons highly regarded in their respective fields of psychiatry, philosophy, and psychology. They collectively make an impressive case for angelic presence. Words spoken by a very wise person over five thousand years ago also seem relevant: Gautama Buddha essentially said, "Do not believe anything, even if I have said it, unless it appeals to your own intelligence." What is left to be done, therefore, rests on the individual decision as one reads this section. While not part of the teachings of Therapeutic Touch, Dora's insights regarding angels and humanity clarify much of the healing experience for the TT therapist of compassionate intent.

A Network of Intelligences

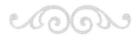

IT IS VERY DIFFICULT TO TALK about the topic of angels, because it is a strange one. I probably have a totally different point of view than most people, who think angels are associated with religion, religious services, and religious belief systems. It is true that angelic presences appear to be accepted in all religious beliefs in the world. However, I think "angels" is a general term at best. Perhaps the designation "intelligences" would be more appropriate to describe the immense scope of their work. They are beings who help to bring about and keep the order in the universe.

To me, order is a natural characteristic. It means, for instance, that trees grow in a certain way: a papaya tree does not suddenly become a pepper tree. Its genetics are part of the constant order relevant to papaya trees, and its relation to humanity is also constant. Angels have to do with humanity, of course, but they also have to do with the balance of Nature. This is an orderly universe because there is communication among these intelligences. The networking that goes on between various consciousnesses is highly complex, but all angelic intelligences agree that there should be an orderly universe.

If you want to understand angels, it is fundamental that you understand the differences between their perspectives and ours. Their sense of time is different; it is really very interesting how different it is. We humans believe ourselves to be bound by birth, life, and death. We have a very narrow sense of time; we calculate it in years, in hours, in moments, and our lives are focused on working our way through time minute by minute. The angels do not think that way. Mountain angels come into physical existence at the beginning of the formation of the mountain and continue with it throughout its existence as a mountain.

They are concerned with time as duration, rather than as the passing of minutes or hours. Their reference is in terms of epochs. However, certain changes do take place, for all things physical undergo change, and change is the basis for our common sense of time passing.

Change in the universe is inevitable, part of the natural evolutionary process. Right now we are in a time of tremendous change due to mass migrations of people, particularly in undeveloped countries. All this human karma is also having a tremendous effect on what happens in Nature. To my perception, the angels do not always like it, but there are some things they cannot alter, such as these extraordinary human migrations. That is human karma; humanity has made the decision, consciously or unconsciously, to migrate, and because of this there are several critical changes arising on our cultural horizons.

When we view war and other power struggles, we think of the universe as disorderly—but who is responsible for this disorder? We humans are. The disorder that is the legacy of human beings manifests in our current disregard of the effects of our interactions with the environment. But in all of the United States, in all of Canada—and I have been in a good many parts of both countries—I think there is a great consciousness and different beings, some of whom I call angels, who establish a certain order. Some of their work is to help huge quantities of people, such as live in New York and other very large cities. There is a great deal of disorder in various cities, but there is also a conscious order helping to keep a balance of subtle energies.

What I am striving to communicate here is this: I don't want you to think of them as duplicates of human beings, because that would be a mistaken impression. Angels have a completely different constitution and makeup than ours. They do not have physical bodies, and they do not have pain, but they do have intelligence and they communicate with one another through the mind. They are on a completely different level of consciousness, and think of the world much more as a unity.

The average human being does not stop to think of the order that pervades the universe, but the angels take that for granted. In today's world the emphasis by far is on destruction. Nobody stresses or is really aware of the order that is all around us. Perhaps scientists understand much more about the sense of order in the universe than do most people.

Still, there has been a change, a reawakening in the United States that was not apparent fifty years ago. People are interested in Nature and its being to an extent unimaginable then. Their minds are not closed to new perspectives as they were then, and the world has significantly changed on many levels. Angels are now a popular topic and we have an unusual opportunity to study them, to try to understand them, and perhaps to make friends with them. As I hope I have made clear, that is not easy, but—in the interest of helping others and with the willingness to exert self-discipline—it can be done.

Several Ways Angels Help Humanity

When there is a substantial disaster, there is an imbalance in Nature. These beings know beforehand that the imbalance will occur, so they are prepared. During the big disasters, many categories of angels come to the scene of the disaster and try to help as much as possible. For the human beings involved, that is their destiny. Many will die; some will be saved by extraordinary means. The various ways the angels help those whose destiny it is to be saved include pouring energy into a person in such a way that they can make their thoughts known. Through a kind of mental telepathy, they give the person ideas about how to help himself, or what he can do to get out of the dangerous predicament. That is, the angels influence a person's mind so he gets an idea that will save him.

Sometimes, but rarely, they have been seen. Angels have helped children, particularly those who are in isolated places and in danger, and several of these children have reported seeing them or their radiance. The angel's duty is to attend to such things—that is, make possible the rescue—and he would obey the tenets of his commitment.

When we need help for ourselves, but particularly when we are reaching out to help others, these beings can, and do, help us. They are in a parallel universe, so to speak, that seems to be invisible to us; however, they do cooperate with us under appropriate circumstances. They help us frequently, and we sense it happening in our uplifted feelings. They have tremendous powers of thought and, among other things, help to keep the balance of many kinds of energy in the world. It is this role that I would stress in discussing them in relation to healing.

Angels and Healing

Healing happens at many different levels, and many different angelic beings are involved in the healing process. They are most prevalent in cases where significant change is involved, such as from birth to life and from life to death, and then they try to help in every way that they can. The way angels help in healing is not a simple thing. As their world is oriented toward a different time frame than ours, they are aware of the future. When they help a human being during times of crisis they do so in a way that will be the most appropriate for the individual's future.

Angels help with the healing interaction, as in Therapeutic Touch, and with the continuing process of healing itself. They help those who wish to help or heal others by assisting in the projection of healing energy to help the ill person attain peace of mind as well as a healing of the physical body. The angels may be able to help people to have peace of mind even when they have pain and are suffering. This peace of mind helps people to have an acceptance, and to grow spiritually.

These beings send harmonizing and healing thoughts to many places where there is great suffering. When people engage in earnest prayers for those who are sick, and they are full of compassion and love for humanity, they draw the attention of healing angels. These angelic beings come to try to help the sufferers, insofar as their karma permits. The angels also help to make the effect as physical as is possible. In the tradition of the laying-on-of-hands, for instance, the healing angels pour their energy through the minister or preacher or dedicated layperson who is conducting the healing service. I find it hard to describe, but the healing angels send energy to the healee's body, enormously increasing the body's own efforts to heal, and accelerating the healing process.

When the great healers of our time, such as Katherine Kuhlman, have healing sessions, the healing angels come to give a blessing to a few of the thousands of people who come. Let me reiterate that *very few* people undergo instantaneous healing. It is the destiny, or karma, of those few to be able to receive that blessing and be healed. In some way the healing angels know which people have the destiny to be healed. Following that knowledge, they pour their energy into the individual's energetic system, and in a few minutes that person is healed. I am convinced that it is not the appeals or the petitions that are critical. It must be the individual's destiny, or it does not happen.

If you are filled with compassion for those who are ill, and if you have—through the sustained centering of your consciousness—a strong intentionality to help them, you are drawing upon this healing power. If you set into motion a healing process such as Therapeutic Touch—in which you center your consciousness, direct your sensitivity to determine where an ill person's energies are not in balance, and then project appropriate vital-energies with intentionality to rebalance the patient's vital-energy field—you can attract these healing angels to help you in the patient's behalf, particularly where large groups are gathered, such as occurs in hospitals. To do this well demands self-discipline of the TT therapist as well as a desire to help. The therapist needs to be emotionally stable in calling on energies of this caliber.

The healing angels focus their energies around structured thoughts such as that of the individual as an intrinsic part of the whole. But if you use a great deal of raw determination and think that what *you* want to do is the right thing—that is, if you get very attached to the results—you will put your ego-directed self in the way of the healing. You will become so involved in having the situation work out *your* way that you will put your anxiety foremost; that is, your anxiety will break into the idea of the patient as whole. When we first started TT we had little children as patients, and the nurses who were learning tried too hard because they wanted the treatment to be successful. However, during the treatment the children cried and got nervous from the tense atmosphere provoked by the nurses. We learned then how important it is to maintain a quiet, peaceful attitude and to remain unattached to the results of our attempts to heal.

Most people think angels will not help people who are dying, but death does not have the same meaning for them as it does for human beings. We human beings think of death in negative terms, but the angels see death from an entirely different perspective. We are very rigid in our ideas, thinking of a lifetime as being limited to three score and ten. They do not think that way; they see a lifetime as an event in a person's soul. On the whole, prayer—good or benign prayer—sends healthy energy to the person to whom the prayer is directed even if he or she is dying. Sometimes when people pray for a person who is very sick, perhaps near death, these beings are there, and they follow that signal. But first of all, they determine whether that person's karma permits a saving intervention.

Particularly in places where many people gather for prayer, there are angels who help during burial services and times of other ceremonials. During the birthing process there is also some angelic presence. They don't interfere in any way, but they are present. It is possible to attract angelic presence through earnest prayer, but, to reiterate, they can do nothing unless that person's karma permits it. Fundamentally, it is not prayer but karma that governs angelic intervention.

It should be kept in mind that in our age particularly it is possible to be saved in a dire emergency by many things: medicine, highly technological means, and other contemporary agencies. Such events can be indicative of destiny, too. From my point of view all significant health interventions have some karmic link; we see karma working itself out every day in hospitals, health agencies, the doctor's office.

Angels and Intentionality

When you specifically focus your attention in the healing act, your mind is open to the ideas and energies of the healing angels. This is one of the avenues open for communication with angels and you can call upon them during the healing interaction. However, it must be for a purpose that is geared to healing others. It is that which draws these forces to you, and you can transmit that powerful healing energy to others. But if you simply go through the motions of healing a person, or do it in a desultory way, the results can be indifferent and without purpose. The committed TT therapist must never think that healing energies or angelic support are there for lackadaisical half-hearted actions.

The energies of the healing angels are available, but drawing their energy demands your active, disciplined engagement in a compassionate act of healing or helping another. For that, you have to lay the groundwork yourself. *It takes mindfulness and discipline to sensitively be quiet for a moment and to transmit angelic healing energies or other kinds of communication with them.* The quiet and the peace are the most important prerequisites. But do not think, "Dear angel, come and help me." Say to yourself, "I am going to help people. Let me touch that force, and I will be quiet so that I can project that sense of peace." If you earnestly direct such a declaration or prayer to the healing angels, they will answer your plea for others' well-being.

If we get an insight suddenly about someone or something, and we can act upon it, then a climate of cooperation and communication with angels can be developed and—if our intuition is sensitive and alert—we can feel whether the interaction was true or not. I personally try to use language carefully when I talk about communication with angels because it puts people off if one uses religious language today. However, when I talk about angels as forces, I am not just using words, I actually believe they are an awesome healing force and that we can call upon their inner linkage with each other when things are at their worst.

An insight does not always depend upon angelic communication. Very often we can get an insight because we are ready, at that moment, to receive that information. We have our own brain, our own intuition. Something within has worked it out for us; not everything is a communication from an angel.

I am interested in two things: healing and the Earth. I am tremendously interested in the environment and Nature, but I also see a great deal of suffering. I am able to be calm and quiet whatever happens, and I have a feeling for what is wrong with a person. I have confidence in my own abilities, so I am not calling upon the angels to help me every minute. It is practice that helps me to gain a greater understanding of Therapeutic Touch. If I want to help a person who is in great pain, then I think of the healing angels as the background for what I do. It never occurs to me to think all the time: "Here is an angel helping me." I just do TT and I know that I can automatically reach out to the universal source of healing energies.

The angels have an impersonality about them because they are helping humankind. They can help anybody very specifically through one of us or through other living beings, but there is a certain impersonality about that interaction. I won't say that having personal interactions such as communications with angels does not happen, but it is rare. As human beings, we want to make everything personal. We want to think that there is a special angel helping us individually, instead of saying: "There are these forces, and if my motive is to want to help, I can draw upon these forces." You will develop your abilities more surely and more strongly if you dedicate your healing work to help suffering humanity.

Angelic Presences During Disasters

There are intelligences that deal with catastrophes and disasters, but how they work may be difficult to understand. Angels that are connected with the Earth use the emotional level of the energies in their auras to sense the feeling of the land as a whole. I think that there is a network of communication between some of these angels, and they know before a disaster strikes. If it is a major natural disaster, something that must happen, a legion of angels would have this knowledge and would be prepared to help.

Disagreement among human beings is inevitable, but with these beings, there is no disagreement, as we understand it. If there are ever any questions, they nevertheless have a recognition that they have a purpose and that they are in touch with a feeling of the land, with a feeling of the future. For instance, just at this time tremendous forest fires are raging in the Northwest, and thousands of acres have been destroyed. To try, even in an inadequate way, to give the perspective of the angels: they experience a sense of loss but they also understand that the trees will grow again as the new seedlings mature, even though it will take fifty or sixty years for the stricken areas to be reforested. The Earth angels have a sense of a constantly changing world and they will put their tremendous energy to the land that is left to foster healthy regrowth. If there is a disaster, they accept it; however, they are concentrated on the future and how their energies can help fulfill that future. We humans have very little of that understanding.

During catastrophic disasters in which many people die, these intelligent beings become very actively involved in helping people as much as they can, but when people die, to them it is not the terrible thing we imagine about death. They see human beings coming into this life, living it, then dying and being reborn, so they have a totally different view of what is happening. However—just as in the healing situations mentioned above—they help all those whose karma permits it. They must be able to see, although I myself cannot, that in the aura of a certain person is some indication that he or she must be saved or given an opportunity to be saved. We hear stories all the time of persons whose lives have been threatened, but then they have a vision of a shining being and they are saved or other versions of that theme. Certain groups, such as the Society of Psychical Research, have kept records of thousands of such cases.

Guardian Angels

There are beings one might call guardian angels; however, I do not think there is one hanging around each person waiting to see what that person will do next. The beings we call guardian angels form a large group but they are not always with a single person. They protect and assist other people too, for their overall job is to help human beings. They do not take care of everybody, but they take on a certain number. If you have a fervent belief in a personal guardian angel, you may think that your guardian angel will help you by preventing you from being murdered, molested, or hurt. But keep in mind that these acts occur by the thousands in the United States alone. There must be thousands upon thousands of people each year who die of accidents or are murdered. According to a simple theory of guardian angels, those persons' guardian angels should have prevented harm from coming to them.

There are beings—they are not quite angels—who try to help certain people. But let me remind you that the critical forces at work in a person's life are dominated by one's karma. A guardian angel, if a person has one, must abide by the person's karmic limitations. If a disaster is going to strike a person, they will help only if it is appropriate. Even if help is given, it may not be as we might see it. In fact, accidental death or even being murdered might be part of a person's karma.

They can, however, help a person to die peacefully. In the case of many of my AIDS patients who have died, for example, we have meditated together for many months, and they have accepted their diagnosis of AIDS. I think that the angels come at the time of their death to give them a special blessing because they have meditated so long and accepted their destiny. Then the dying process goes very peacefully. This doesn't happen if the person fights his dying, but it does if the person is accepting. The angels try to help those who are not accepting of death, but they are not so successful at these times.

One's spiritual acceptance of such occurrences is how inner growth takes place. In this regard I think of the AIDS patients in our Seattle healing group who help me as I work on various other patients. It is difficult to imagine how profoundly this privilege of helping another in need transfigures them. They have accepted their dying, they are very peaceful, and because they themselves have been affected, they give their all while doing Therapeutic Touch to other patients. It helps them have confidence in their inner self, that epitome of personal order. Once more I will stress that angels are part of Nature and its order, for upon that recognition depends a valid understanding of angels.

The Earth Angels

One category within the angelic domain is that of the Earth angels who have their roots of consciousness in whatever land or mountains are within their sphere of concern. With that intelligence they not only maintain a certain order, they also do whatever is necessary to keep that land alive. They are oriented toward changes that are important to the well-being of Nature herself, such as changes in temperature or humidity. The Earth angels' auras and consciousness are sensitive to many miles of countryside, but of course they are not especially sensitive to each individual being in that territory. They relate to the welfare of all life within that ecological niche, including the animals, trees, and plants, as a group consciousness.

In themselves, they have nothing to do with human beings. In fact, there are often few or no human beings in their areas; throughout the world there are vast stretches of mountains and land where human beings rarely come. But when human beings are present, they become part of the angels' general concern.

When we can spend large amounts of time outdoors, it is not difficult to realize that we are part of Nature. Realizing that wild animals are a natural part of this relationship also and acting toward them in a manner that elicits a sense of trust will also bring us closer to the angelic beings who sense the unity of all living creatures.

The Angel of the Grand Canyon

A very unique intelligence oversees the region of the Grand Canyon, a magnificent spectacle and great tourist attraction that has been preserved by the government. The canyon itself is an immense chasm reaching down through ageless strata of multicolored rock to a river flowing below. It is very interesting that there is a very strong angelic being there who has an intensely determined sense of wanting to protect not only the canyon itself, but also the land around it. The Angel of the Grand Canyon is incredibly beautiful. Physically, it is very craggy. When I first went there it gave me a tremendous feeling of strength and a completely different sense of the fundamental character of the United States.

This Earth angel is also very protective toward the American Indians whose land surrounds the Grand Canyon. Many years ago, I stayed for two summers in New Mexico. I got to know some of the Indians and went to the pueblos, some of which are over a thousand years old. During that time, I got to know some of the Indian leaders and also some of the members of Congress who fought for the American Indians. Several, I felt, were truly inspired by the angelic presence in those lands.

In that area one gets a feeling that is unique because the interaction between the angels and humans finds its roots in another time, in another tradition. The people, themselves, are different: they have a strong sense of Nature and identification with Nature, and their thinking is molded by this singular relationship. I am not an American Indian, and I think I might do them an injustice in trying to explain their relationship with the angelic kingdom. However, I suppose they have a greater kinship to the feelings and perspective of these expressions of Nature.

Mountains and Angelic Presence

There is also a special intelligence in great mountains. Mountains exist for a long time; they are very stable on the whole, and the angelic beings associated with mountains are, in general, very strong. When I look out of the front door of my home in Seattle, I see a whole chain of mountains. They are snow-capped part of the year and rise tall and majestic. They are constantly in the process of change, but they have been there for thousands of years; they endure, and it is that ability to endure in the face of change that is striking.

To most people, the distinctive intelligence of each mountain feels different from that of others. If you climb mountains, your relation to them becomes more personal, and the individual distinctions between these beings become more meaningful and apparent. When I was young I lived near many volcanoes. They are part of the consciousness of a mountain. They are both of the Earth and the element of fire, so they have a very different consciousness. When there are volcanic eruptions, a great deal of land is destroyed as well as living creatures being put in jeopardy, and widespread changes may result. The Earth angels get signals ahead of time about future events, so they get a sense that something is going to happen. I do not say that they like or don't like what is about to happen but that they accept change. There is nothing they can do about it, but they can, and do, help in every way. Therefore they can be very stable influences during such times.

Angels of the Seas

I have traveled widely and have seen the angels of the seas, natural beings in the oceans of the world. Their territory is enormous, encompassing thousands of miles. They have a different intelligence than the Earth or land angels but they maintain an active network of communication with them. Life in the sea is complicated in itself and has a distinctly different atmosphere than that of the land. It is a natural life devoid of much interference from human beings, and this contributes to the difference between the angels of the seas and the angels of the land. The angels of the seas have a consciousness that affects living beings, and they do affect the Earth, for they are as much a part of it as the land angels. I do not think they are very evolved, in a certain sense, because they do not deal with difficulties of the degree that human beings do. They do, however, engage in disasters throughout the world; in fact, many natural disasters take place in the oceans of the world. If there are tremendous storms, this intelligence is exchanged with the land angels before the landfall of the disastrous storm.

The Angel of New York

The Angel of New York City is remarkable, with an enormous sphere of influence. He is big in every sense of the word: he covers a large territory and he is a very evolved being. He encompasses millions of people who are doing diverse things: loving and hating, sometimes committing acts of violence, sometimes going to church and portraying great acts of faith. All this and more happens daily in an atmosphere in flux. For forty-one years I lived just outside New York and commuted into the city frequently. From my point of view, this great consciousness has the charge to keep peace in spite of all the violence, all the different beliefs and opinions of the people of New York. The streams of strong human emotions that are constantly being poured out are ultimately assisted towards a dynamic energetic balance by this being.

New York City itself is part of his aura; through this medium, all positive thoughts are used to keep the whole flux in balance. For instance, the moment there is significant violence in one part of New York, the Angel of New York is aware of it and helps to distribute some of the more constructive and positive human energies from another part of New York to balance out the emotional atmosphere of the city. When people in New York meditate or gather in a church and think of peace and send it out, some of that energy is used by the angel to keep a balance in thought and action among all living creatures in the city.

Other angels function in New York, too. There are churches, synagogues, and other religious places that attract angels concerned with the outpouring of faith and aspiration. When people go to these religious centers and have a deep intent to align themselves with the philosophy and ceremonies of their particular faith, they pray and sing its praises.

On holidays the attendance is in the hundreds and perhaps in the thousands in places. As that expression of devotion is raised to their highest ideals, two things can happen: the attraction of angels, and the addition of their blessing, or their energy, to that of the congregation. The angels send helpful thoughts to these people and pour their healing energy into them to help them feel unified and to give them extra energy at that time. The angels are also able to use the enormous goodwill of the members of the congregation.

The Angel of New York City, together with the other angels, distributes those uplifting feelings throughout New York to those who are receptive to them. The purpose of this is to help to maintain balance, particularly in places that are in need of that stability and sense of equanimity. Although rarely noticed or realized, this subtle balancing goes on continually.

If we could appreciate that there is such a balancing process available, it would be much easier to live in big cities. It is important to know that we can make some contribution. All of us who are consciously sending out a healing energy, and with it a sort of meditation, add to the balance of order in a place. When we meditate on sending thoughts of peace to the world, our combined efforts do help. We all can help in this work with our meditations, prayers, and affirmations and in a physical way as well. By doing this we are not so much helping the angels as we are helping the rest of humanity. It is thrilling to realize that if you consciously exert your intentionality to send thoughts of peacefulness and quietness to those in turmoil, you can help the angels in their efforts toward an atmosphere of equanimity and harmony among all living beings.

I do this when I travel, for I know that it helps the emotional ambience of the place I am in and the country at large. Every night when I go to bed in a different city, I think of this. It makes it easier for me to feel at home in a place. If we ourselves are in difficulty, it will help if we keep in mind that there are beings who—although we cannot see them—have our welfare at heart. Then it will be easier to believe in an orderly universe.

Angels of Music and Sound

Music and sound come under the province of a special worldwide class of angels who inspire a high degree of music appreciation in all people, particularly those who have a deep feeling for music. These angels come to concerts and other musical performances and help to inspire both the performers and the audiences. While they work most frequently with large groups of people, I think that small groups of people who were dedicated to music might also draw them. I think that persons can get in touch with the angels of sound if the desire to communicate with them is genuine.

Sound has a very special effect upon people, perhaps more than we realize. Think for a moment about the stirring effects of national anthems. Whether you like them or not, the sound of the music has a powerful effect upon those who hear them. In various cultures sound and music are different, but I think that in all cultures music and sound express what is *inside* a culture. The times when people come together to enjoy music are important events. I spent my early childhood in Java, a predominantly Muslim country where, strangely, the story of Krishna in the Bhagavad Gita was often enacted, accompanied with musical instruments, before huge audiences. I listened to that throughout my childhood, as did millions and millions of other people of that culture. I think it had a very fine effect, for these angels of sound came; they helped to distribute the uplifting effect of this inspiring story among the people and they participated energetically in those mass meetings.

I think the same thing happens in the United States in places such as Tanglewood, the summer music camp of the Boston Symphony Orchestra. Thousands of people attend the rehearsals and the performances that are held there throughout the summer. There are special angels who are present at large concerts, such as Tanglewood, and they also try to help persons who are engaged in evolving new concepts of music.

Being Sensitive to Angelic Presence

If you wish to understand angelic life, the first principle is to look closely at what is happening around you. Keen observations of natural happenings open one's mind and make one sensitive to these beings. This may seem a peculiar thing for me to say, but we are usually so unaware of most things around us that we don't even notice physical things adequately. We take things for granted without really appreciating what they are. So look and then, perhaps, look again; try to understand the place of particular events in the scheme of things, try to see them in proportion and context. Such focused awareness may sound like a burdensome chore, but I find it fun to be keenly observant. I don't know how many times I have driven across this country in a car, from east to west and west to east, and many directions in between. I have always been interested in what I perceive and I take great pleasure in seeing the trees or green foliage, but I also note the condition of the trees and the plants and make a judgment about how they are thriving or what care they might need. But most people in our culture do not take their leisure in natural surroundings where they can passively watch what is happening around them.

Another strange thing I might say is that by being open and observant and sensitive to a place, we can become aware and understand something about what angels are expressing by their thoughts. We can get ideas in many different ways. For instance, both intellectual and emotional problems respond to such a nonaggressive atmosphere. The person involved finds he suddenly can relax and in this moment an unexpected intuition about the problem can occur. In this way—by the conscious use of our feelings or our minds—we can get in touch with these beings.

I don't think you can involve an angel to help you when you have lost a pocketbook, a pen, or any other physical object. Why would they care? That's a particularly human problem. When you pray to find your pocketbook you are quiet for a moment and perhaps your own intuition flashes on its whereabouts; I do not think angelic help is part of it. In other words, one should not attribute every personal event to angelic intervention.

However, if you really want to help or heal human beings, that is a different thing. Those interactions involve living organisms and there are angels who are connected to living organisms, to Nature, and all it implies. Without a doubt, when you want to help, cooperation and communication are very possible. That communication might in fact occur if you really search and have a strong desire for it. You can reach the sort of energy that is characteristic of angelic communication when you are genuinely trying to help Nature, or when you are helping people. But you have to be willing to exert self-discipline to create the necessary conditions of quiet within and cultivate a dedicated and sensitive awareness to what is occurring around you.

Communicating with Angels

The trouble about communicating with angels is us. We are so often locked up in our own thoughts and our own habit patterns, and the beings that we call angels do not think like human beings. Most human beings rarely feel a part of the universe, but the angels play an intrinsic role in that dynamism because of their sensitivity. Although some people have a sense that they have a part in the dynamics of the universe, they get very involved in their life activities and they don't consciously engage in it as intelligent humans beings. Angels have bigger horizons; they recognize that they are fundamentally linked as part of the order of the universe.

When we think of our world, we think of where we are at the moment, or where we are in the United States, but we may not think of ourselves in relation to the universe, as part of a universal scheme. But the angels see and participate in the fundamental order underlying all the disorder. All aspects of the universe take part in that universal principle of order whether the scope of activity is related to the birthing of stars or to human birth, life, or death.

This is automatically part of the consciousness of all the angelic orders; this is perhaps the most significant difference between the angels and ourselves. It underlies their acceptance and their belief systems and gives them a fundamentally different perspective than ours. Consequently their relationship to humanity occurs at a different level of consciousness than that which frames our usual outlook on life and defines our everyday reality. The context of their relationship to humanity occurs most naturally at that level of consciousness that we call the inner self, the deeper level where we are all tied together in consciousness.

Of course, they think that human beings are funny, because they do not understand our motivations. Sometimes what we do is bewildering to their sense of what is happening. For instance, I do not think they understand the origin of our violent feelings when we blow up over some emotional issue. Still, they try to balance these impassioned energies, for that is their commitment.

When we think of communication, we usually think of it occurring by talking and listening, by reading and writing, or by intently listening to music or other coded sounds. But in special instances, communication can occur through meditation or silence in which there is a meeting of minds and a sense of peace pervades. It is at those times that we can visualize a reaching out from within Nature itself and an extension of that sense of peace to others. Let us take the experience of attending a concert. You sit together with others who also like music and, if you respond to the music, it has a focusing and unifying effect on your emotions and your thoughts. It evokes within you a different sense of being and a feeling of togetherness with all in the concert hall.

However, communication within the angelic kingdom is a very difficult concept to grasp because it is so different from our usual experience. It does not occur by doing; it is concerned with how the angelic beings affect our minds and emotions. *It is not language per se that makes it happen; it is the mind.* That is how we communicate with them and how they communicate with one another. It is hard for us to imagine but the following conception is close to what happens in their communications: if I could think very clearly about ideas and make pictures in my mind about them, this could be perceived by angelic forces. This is not exact, but it conveys that their communication is not in language; *it is in being able to clearly project the ideas behind words.*

To experience this you have to encourage a deep sense of quiet within yourself. The sustained centering of consciousness is not only very important in meditation and the Therapeutic Touch process, it is also an essential tool in accurately communicating with angels. In daily life our minds are full of how we are going to solve the problems of the moment; most of our lives are spent in that way. Sometimes even five minutes of quietness—particularly when we are troubled, when we do not know the right thing to do—will help us to get a sense of this inner communication. If you can become very quiet within yourself when you have questions or problems and you are worried about them, that is the moment when the minds of these beings can be reached. But quiet or stillness is essential.

Let me tell you a story that illustrates how all angelic orders communicate their thoughts to one another and how they influence humanity. One day Dolores and I held a group healing meditation. One of our participants had a mother in a hospital over one hundred miles away, and so we did healing at a distance for the mother. The mother had been in a very fractious state of mind, her blood pressure was considerably elevated, she was very uncomfortable, frightened, and unstable, and her daughter was concerned.

The healing meditation includes certain aspects of Therapeutic Touch in which you clearly visualize yourself at the bedside of the patient doing TT. You then treat the patient as may seem necessary from the assessment. The whole group did this healing meditation for her and sent her thoughts of quietness and peace.

About an hour and a half later her daughter phoned the hospital to find out how her mother was doing. They said that something very remarkable had occurred. She had been in a dangerous state: her blood pressure had risen uncontrollably, she was very restive, and considerably upset emotionally. But suddenly there had been a decided change in her state of consciousness and she quietly and peacefully went into a deep sleep. When she awoke, her blood pressure and other vital signs were completely normal and she said she felt well rested.

I tell this story to emphasize that thought—particularly clear thoughts guided by intentionality—can have a significant effect on a person even some distance away. Of course the members of this group were practiced meditators, one of whom was personally concerned. All these are conditions that would facilitate the process, particularly the concern of the daughter, which guided our thoughts to her mother. This is how angels communicate, not by talking, but by the clear projection of thoughts and feelings. In our desire to help those in need, we can become sensitive to angelic presence and to their means of communications. We can nurture that possibility by maintaining openness to nonordinary means of communication and to alternate perspectives of life and living. This entails a sustained self-discipline that fosters a clarity of thought and a recognition that we never need feel ourselves alone.

Positive and Negative Energies

On the whole, angels use positive energies and try to dissipate negative energies. I do not think they can change negative energies instantly, but they can disperse that energy and thereby weaken its effects. If they did not dissipate such energies, it is possible that the memory of these negative energies in certain places could continue for several weeks.

I think there are negative forces in the world, but I avoid the terms "evil" and "good" because they represent extremes, absolute opposites that exclude everything else. I like to speak of positive and negative energies. There are negative beings but I would not call them angels. To get a sense of what I mean, can you admit that there is a great deal of violence and greed in the world? These negative beings get their strength from the negative emotions that humanity produces. They actually feed on them. In a place like New York City there is a concentration of both positive and negative human energies. They do not battle in the ordinary sense of the word, but the Angel of New York and other positive angels try to pour out positive energy when they find there is a concentration of negative energies in the territory or area for which they are responsible. That is their job, and they are committed to it.

When people congregate in a certain part of a city, the angels would spend more time balancing that particular area. As I mentioned, there is an active, working relationship among the different kinds of angels. In New York City one community effort that might form a nucleus for such relationship is the coalitions of neighborhoods that have come together to turn burned-out vacant lots into beautiful, healthy gardens where vegetables and flowers are grown during the spring and summer months. Such opportunities for mutual interaction are most encouraging.

Today, in the United States, there seem to be two factions concerned with the environment. One, which is made up primarily of young people, is very strongly concerned with the protection of the environment. The other group consists mostly of people who want to use the environment for their own special purposes. There is a struggle going on between the two groups. Some people feel very discouraged, but young people seem to be spreading the idea of a need and responsibility to protect the environment, particularly to others of their generation throughout the world. Such actions give one hope that things will change. The intensity of unconcerned, rather mindless, destruction of rain forests and pollution of the waterways is already lessening to a significant degree, and that is encouraging. These struggles are not over, and there will be constant changes, but the level of intelligent concern and action is heartening.

Consciousness is working through different intelligences in the invisible world, who inhabit that world and function through it, whether we are aware of them or not. This recognition should make us feel safer: that there are beings who are participating in keeping the order in Nature, who try to help humanity while also helping the Earth to keep stable. However, the objectives of our industrial empires often conflict with them. Nevertheless, who thought fifty years ago that Congress would pass a law restricting the cutting down of trees? It is a tremendous accomplishment that now a law has been passed to conserve tree life. I do not believe in exaggerating, so I must be careful of my words. However, I was wondering whether all this recent mind-change has been influenced by the angels. The world *has* changed for the good, in many instances, and part of humanity has worked mightily to support that change. What I would like you to remember from this discussion is that the part the angels play in their interactions with humanity is that of significantly affecting the minds of people.

Questions and Answers

Question: *Have you seen angels personally?*

Yes, of course. I've been able to see them since I was quite young. I'm not talking out of the back of my head because I have read a book! Most of what I am telling you is from my personal experience. I know what I am saying; I've never kept it a secret, have I? But I don't talk very much about it.

Question: *What do they look like?*

It depends upon what kind they are. Some of the ones that deal with human beings may have a human face or part of them may be human-like; and they are surrounded by big, shining auras. I suppose that the idea of wings arose in people's minds because of the shining of their auras. Also, wings are a symbol of spirituality, particularly in Christianity. In other religions, for instance, Hinduism, they do believe in beings or intelligences such as devas or angels, but they do not necessarily have wings.

I think of angels as consciousnesses that can be simultaneously aware of more things than we can. For example, they can be constantly sensitive about *all* the people in a room. We all are conscious, but—if you look back at your own experience—you will realize that you do not have this *total awareness*. If an angel came into a room with you, he would become sensitive to what you are feeling; he would actually see what you are feeling. We look at the physical first, but an angel would look at what you are thinking and feeling. He would not be interested whether you are thin, fat, green, or purple. He would be interested in your consciousness. Certain angels—not all—would know something about your destiny. The ones who were highly evolved would pick this up, and the healing angels, without any doubt, would know about your sickness and destiny.

Question: *Have angels ever lived in a physical body, like human beings do?*

Well, a lot of people think so. I don't, but there is a vast literature on that subject. However, I never have had that experience. I think there is a special evolvement and a special energy being brought in at this time; beyond that I cannot say.

Question: *Do angels die?*

Not in the way we do; however, eventually it is time for them to go. They live much longer than we do. The particular thing that they have come to do is finished, and their consciousness also disappears, but of course they have no physical body. They transform and go on to other things; that is, their consciousness takes another form. It is not a birth as we know it in the physical world, but another aspect or attribute of consciousness in which they inhere.

Question: *You refer to angels as "he." Are angels in fact masculine or feminine energy?*

I think they are both, and some of them do not have gender. The highest angels are neither male nor female.

Question: *If you wanted to communicate with angels, would it be with emotion or thought?*

Thoughts and emotions would be the avenue I would take, and they would pick it up immediately.

Question: *Can humans understand their communication?*

Yes, I think we can. They can either communicate by visual images or their thoughts can assume our language structure. We don't hear it in words, but in ideas. If they help people they do not speak in so many words, but they put ideas in one's head. For instance, they will forcibly put a thought or idea in a person's mind to guide him out of danger, giving the person a clear sense of: I have to do this thing and then that thing.

Question: *Would angels be present at moments of great creativity such as when a composer or artist is creating a great masterpiece?*

They might have some influence, but I don't think they will sit behind the back of a person all the time. I think that when a person feels inspired, they may contact him or her in thought and in this way give these ideas more reality. I think they can feed inspired persons with ideas and energy.

Question: *Do you think that angels work through people who do Therapeutic Touch?*

They could, in cases of emergency, for instance. Not during a routine healing, however.

Question: *Do angels ever take human form?*

As I said, to *us* they have a human form. They don't quite look like us, although they do have a somewhat human form. But, I think there is a different quality about them. We have our wrinkles and other imperfections. They can have a human form; however, they do not interact with the environment in the same way we do, nor do their faces reflect emotional strain and turmoil as ours do.

Question: *If a person moves to a different neighborhood, does their guardian angel go with them, or do they get a different angel?*

I don't know. I travel a lot and I say "Hi!" to a lot of angels! Some angels are related to particular sites and they remain at that site. Guardian angels don't have to travel as we do. For myself, in every city I travel to, I always take a few minutes and think of the angels and reach out to them. I travel all over the world, but I always consciously go out to them in whatever city I am in. And it is nice to feel "at home" in different places.

Question: *Do angels have different personalities?*

They do have different personalities. They also are different than are our expectations. When I go to a place, I pick up angels of a different personality or a different outlook, and I think that makes life much more exciting.

Question: *Do you have names for the angels you talk to?*

No, I don't. I travel so much, and only stay at a few places for some time.

Question: *You mentioned that the Earth angels watch over the wild animals in their areas in groups during disasters. What about pets?*

I am not sure that this relationship is clear to me. In my family, we have a cat whom we all adore. This is an old cat. If a disaster occurs I don't know whether or not the cat would be closer to the human being and follow the human's signals, and thus not be so open to the angelic forces. In the wilderness, the animals respond to a group consciousness. I don't know whether a cat that has been so domesticated would respond in the same way. I think it would have lost that sense of communion with wild animals, but it would turn toward the human element in its life. It is an interesting thought, one I had never considered before. On the other side, there are many stories of pets knowing of disasters before they occurred and warning their human friends, or leading them to safety, sometimes even if it endangers themselves.

Question: *Is there one angel that oversees the campsites at Pumpkin Hollow or Indralaya?*

The angels work very much on a universal level. Beings such as angels do not "belong" to a circumscribed site alone. They are not necessarily everywhere, but I think they are in places such as Pumpkin Hollow and Indralaya where Nature is unspoiled. The atmosphere enables the people in that area to be a little closer to the sense of belonging to Nature. And the angels particularly relate to areas where humans have made an informed and concerted effort to be in touch with them. Knowing that there are people who are striving to understand the angelic kingdom draws the attention of angels who relate to that area.

If you think about them, I think you will draw their attention, because you are really in a unique place. I don't think anyone in one hundred miles or more talks like we do about the intelligent beings. We talk about angels and meditate on angels, so we are outstanding in this consciousness. They think of us as a group of people who know something about them. Besides, we have a strong feeling for the environment. I think when we sit by the waterfall or other quiet places in camp, we really go out in a sense of unity with Nature. They realize this and so they appreciate us in every way.

Some of these beings are fairies, many of which do not affect human beings at all; they have their own lives, somewhat like mice, you might say. They are entities who do not have too much intelligence, but they are also part of this invisible life net in Nature. They are part of the harmonies in the cascading water of the stream and part of the garden. They exist to help Nature, and they are a part of the world of the Earth angels. Basically, they have little to do with humanity; their work is with plants and the angelic consciousness of Earth.

If you work in the garden, you have an opportunity to set up a relationship with them. They will like you, but they are not going to heal you. They are friendly. If you want to grow a plant nobody thinks will grow, love it and ask these fairies, "Help me," and they will help you. They like growing things. Don't do this because you want to be unique, but because it is an interesting experiment. People have succeeded in doing that. However, the angels have a much deeper relationship to humanity because humans are part of the big issues of the world, whereas fairies belong to the world of growing things in Nature.

Question: *Are there any angels here, now?*

Well, around us, some of them are. Yes, sure.

Question: *Do angels have a sense of humor?*

I think they do—we are having fun right now on supposedly such a serious subject! I think they like the sound of laughter, and it is very healthy for us to laugh.

Afterword

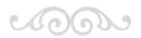

It has taken Dora and me over thirty years to put together the complex healing process we call Therapeutic Touch, and neither of us ever declared its formation to be complete. Rather, we recognized that Therapeutic Touch is intrinsically based upon the constitution of human beings, many fundamental aspects of which continue to be not well understood, even in modern times. Insights into the TT process, therefore, will continue to grow naturally with future generations of perceptive persons who are compassionately concerned with helping and healing those in need. Nevertheless, Dora's sensitive regard for those who are ill, in crisis, or undergoing trauma, and her penetrating wisdom about the subtle energy dynamics of those conditions has cut a wide swath in our ignorance and underlies much of the credence with which Therapeutic Touch is viewed today.

Dora was always reticent to talk about her personal life. She became quite adept at putting off those who were too curious about her unique perceptual abilities with a simple, soft answer, and used her high-spirited, effervescent laughter, her considerable wit, and her impressive wisdom to ease out of such confrontations. There is, in fact, a biography on her in progress at this time, which will give voice to the broad scope of her many accomplishments. However, it is appropriate to include here a brief record of her several seminal contributions to the fuller understanding of the healing process, upon which she focused the last thirty years of her life.

Dora had a complex personality that was anchored in pragmatic common sense. This aspect of her life found expression for more than a decade through her work as president of a large national organization, and as director on the board of a national corporation that developed innovative teaching methods and materials for primary education in mathematics. Her exceptional development of her special perceptual faculties made her a much sought-after consultant, particularly among medical scientists in psychiatry, psychosomatic medicine, neurology, and oncology, and among clinicians concerned with multiple sclerosis, as well as for people with AIDS, cancer, and Alzheimer's and Parkinson's syndromes.

She was widely read and had a deep and longtime interest in much of the current medical research being done, particularly in the areas noted above. It was most interesting to see how Dora could reflect in her own studies a close approximation ("approximation" because her perspective was so different than that of traditional medicine) of the control, unbiased conditions, and insistence on repeated trials that are core requirements in the scientific method. Conforming to these standards, she made at least two original findings that I know of. First, during a series of studies that focused on patients with psychosomatic symptoms, she found a previously unknown, very small coccygeal gland that operates near the base of the spine. More recently, during a study of persons with fibromyalgia and chronic pain syndrome, Dora located a nonphysical area in the left parietal region of the brain that was common to a majority of these people. Neither of these sites have been given formal recognition by medical science to date. She came upon other rare findings in her studies of the chakras of patients of the neuropsychiatrist, Shafica Karagulla (Karagulla and Kunz, 1989), as mentioned in Section IV: Chakras and the Therapeutic Touch Process. Several of her books, including *The Chakras and the Human Energy Field*, have become classics in their fields.

Dora was also an excellent role model as a compassionate healer. The major part of her life was dedicated to meeting with ill people, wherever she was in the world, to discuss with them their conditions from her point of view, that is, from the perspective of the dynamics of the subtle energies involved. She would do Therapeutic Touch with them and suggest "homework"—practices or behavioral changes that might be helpful to them. She never accepted money for her healing work, nor did she for the many lectures and workshops on Therapeutic Touch that she gave to professional persons in hospitals, universities, and private agencies. She often met with health professionals and offered them suggestions and critique on how they could become more sensitive to the needs of their clients. In particular, her work was the basis of several innovative changes, especially in the care of those in psychiatric centers, at agencies for persons with AIDS, and in hospices.

Dora was concerned with healthy people as well as with those who were ill. She was very attentive to the future of society and the role those who are now children would play, specifically the many highly sensitive children that have come among us today. Another aspect of her work, therefore, was meeting with such children and their parents, counseling with them and sharing her uncommon insights.

In all, Dora was one-of-a-kind, and this exceptional lady lent Therapeutic Touch a singular reflection of what we can do to help those in need, and what we can do to help ourselves fulfill a most humane aspect of our being. Dora, therefore, is an exemplary model in the history of Therapeutic Touch.

What, however, of its future? Since its inception, Therapeutic Touch has been spreading worldwide and, of course, it will change with the times. TT was called into being to meet the problems of people who were ill, in trauma or crisis, or in final transition, but whose needs were not being met by traditional medical care. For a large segment of the world's population, these needs are still unfulfilled. Because of this, the need for a valid alternative continues, a need that can be excellently met by Therapeutic Touch.

Moreover, the future consumers of healing will have new illnesses and traumas called out by our concerted worldwide allowance of persistent changes in the planet's natural environment, which have been coupled with new modes of living with synthetic materials. As recent research has demonstrated, these are problems that can be alleviated by intervention with the Therapeutic Touch process. TT treatment is also well equipped to address the fatigue, anxiety, and stress that are being intensified by high-tech living. There is still another area that will demand the attention of future researchers into the possibilities of TT treatment: that of preventing or confronting the health problems laypeople will be exposed to unwittingly by the heedless rush to develop ever-new energy sources whose long term use has not been adequately studied, such as the recent replacement of petroleum by hydrogen as fuel.

On a brighter note, I feel quite certain that a positive use of Therapeutic Touch in future will occur within both the nuclear and the extended family. It is being used in this way now to a growing extent and some encouraging reports are in. For instance, its practice lends itself to enhancing insights into previously little understood problems of family members, as well as to deeper bonding within the family, as a sharpening of perceptions about relationships has occurred among them.

This array of possible needs for therapeutic intervention is diverse. However, Therapeutic Touch responds favorably to an unusually broad spectrum of ailments, as is compellingly demonstrated by its history. It is that very ability to be sensitive to a large number of conditions that fortifies a belief that Therapeutic Touch will continue to be versatile in the future to help and to heal those in need.

To Dora, with Love

When we think of you, Dora
our minds remember your laughter
its spontaneous quality
its contagious nature
how it bubbled out
issued forth from a heart
warmed and brimming with compassion.

You were most your Self
when caring for those in need
wholeheartedly tending
for those struck down
or those just stuck.
You challenged
everyone you knew
to see life
to live their life
"Can I say this"
—you'd say with your white head
cocked to the side

and with one eye half-squinted—
from a new perspective.
"You see what I'm saying."

Your energy sprang,
almost leaped at times,
from an almost
inexhaustible fount
it was measured
within your being
then shared with gems
of practical wisdom
coming from the true heart
of a truly "Practical Girl
—who lived a crazy life."

Dora, you truly
lived a life dedicated to giving
dedicated to serving
and although we'll miss
your grace—
the gifts you shared
will be realized ages hence
when we too
can glimpse through
nature's inner veil
and join your dedicated quest
for a farther shore.

Your therapeutic touch
touched us in so many ways
over many years
through many ills
and even though we know
in our hearts
you still linger just out of reach

we'll miss your
echoing peals of laughter—
laughter
that still lurks
that still lives
just beyond our touch
in the swaying of the wind
or a babble from a brook—
it's a sound to listen for
hidden in nature
and alive within the hug
of one's favorite tree.

—charlie elkind 8/25/99

References

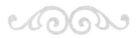

Books by Dora Kunz and Dolores Krieger

Karagulla, Shafica and Dora Kunz. 1989. *The Chakras and the Human Energy Field*. Wheaton, Ill: Quest Books.

Krieger, Dolores. 1979. *The Therapeutic Touch: How to Use Your Hands to Help or to Heal*. Englewood Cliffs, N.J.: Prentice-Hall, Inc.

——————. 1981. *Foundations of Holistic Health Nursing Practices: The Renaissance Nurse*. Philadelphia: JB Lippincott.

——————. 1987. *Living the Therapeutic Touch: Healing as a Lifestyle*. New York: Dodd, Mead and Co.

——————. 1993. *Accepting Your Power to Heal: The Personal Practice of Therapeutic Touch*. Santa Fe, N. Mex.: Bear & Company.

——————. 1997. *Therapeutic Touch Inner Workbook: Ventures in Transpersonal Healing*. Santa Fe, N. Mex.: Bear & Company.

——————. 2002. *Therapeutic Touch As Transpersonal Healing*. New York: Lantern Books.

Kunz, Dora, ed. 1986. *Spiritual Aspects of the Healing Arts*. Wheaton, Ill.: Quest Books.

Kunz, Dora van Gelder. 1991. *The Personal Aura*. Wheaton, Ill.: Quest Books.

——————. 1977. *The Real World of Fairies*. Wheaton, Ill.: Quest Books.

Other Works Cited

Fry, Christopher. 1951. *A Sleep of Prisoners*. London: Oxford University Press.

Grof, Stanislav. 1988. Modern Consciousness Research and Human Survival. In *Human Survival and Consciousness Evolution*, ed. S. Grof. Albany, N.Y.: State University of New York Press.

Houston, Jean. 1993. *Life Force: The Psycho-Historical Recovery of the Self*. Wheaton, Ill: Quest Books.

Tart, Charles. 1981. Transpersonal realities or neurophysiological realities? In *Metaphors of Consciousness*, ed. Ronald S. Valle and Rolf von Eckarsberg. New York: Plenum Press.

Wilber, Ken. 1980. *The Atman Project*. Wheaton, Ill.: Quest Books.

Therapeutic Touch
Resources

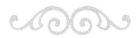

The Official Organization of Therapeutic Touch:
Nurse Healers - Professional Associates, International
3760 South Highland Drive, Suite #429
Salt Lake City, Utah 84106
Phone: 801-273-3399
Email: NH-PAI@therapeutic-touch.org
Fax: 901-273-3352

Long-term Courses in Therapeutic Touch:
Pumpkin Hollow Foundation
1184 Route 11
Craryville, New York 12521
Phone: 518-325-3583
Email: pumpkin@taconic.net
Fax: 518-325-5633

Orcas Island Foundation
360 Indralaya Road
Eastsound, Washington 98245
Email: oif@rockland.com
Fax: 360-376-5977

Therapeutic Touch Network of Ontario
123 Queen Street
Brampton, ON, Canada L6Y 1M3
Phone: 905-454-2688
Email: Marydale@idirect.com
Fax: 905-453-3747

Index